What is narrative therapy?

An easy-to-read introduction

by

Alice Morgan

DULWICH CENTRE PUBLICATIONS

ADELAIDE   SOUTH AUSTRALIA

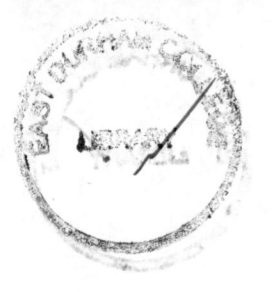

Copyright © 2000 *by* Dulwich Centre Publications
ISBN 0 9577929 0 5

published by
Dulwich Centre Publications
Hutt St PO Box 7192
Adelaide, South Australia 5000
phone (61-8) 8223 3966 fax (61-8) 8232 4441
email: dcp@senet.com.au
www.dulwichcentre.com.au

The views expressed in this book are not necessarily those of the Publisher.
No part of this book may be reproduced or transmitted by any process
whatsoever without the prior written permission of the Publisher.

Printed & manufactured in Australia by:
Graphic Print Group, Richmond, South Australia

Contents

A note from the publisher

This book seeks to introduce people to the ideas and ways of working that have come to be known as narrative therapy. We specifically asked Alice Morgan to reproduce the ideas of others here in an easy to read introduction.

The ideas and ways of working contained in this book were introduced to the therapy realm by David Epston and Michael White. Their versions of this work can be found within a wide range of books and articles, which they have written. Over the last ten years, a variety of other therapists have engaged with narrative practices and have made significant contributions to what is a constantly evolving body of knowledge and skills.

For those of you who find this book interesting, we strongly recommend that you follow up the references that are included at the end of various chapters. Within these books or articles you will find the original descriptions of the ideas that Alice is introducing here. You will also find thorough articulations of the thinking that informs narrative practice.

For now though, we are very pleased to welcome you to this easy-to-read introduction which, as its title suggests, seeks to answer the question: What is narrative therapy?

Acknowledgements

This project began due to the idea and invitation of Cheryl White and was sustained through her continual interest and encouragement. After receiving the invitation and taking a deep breath, Alice Morgan wrote an initial draft of this book, which David Denborough worked on before it was then distributed to a wide range of people for feedback and suggestions. Those who were able to offer feedback included Maggie Carey, Loretta Perry, Shona

Russell, Jan Tonkin, Rose Barnes, Carol Trowbridge and Michael White. After receiving their ideas, feedback and examples, David Denborough and Alice Morgan worked thoroughly on the draft, which travelled back and forth from Melbourne to Adelaide (thank goodness for email!) until it came into its current form. Jane Hales was responsible for the layout and Melissa Raven for proof reading. Alice would also like to acknowledge the influence that her teachers have had on her therapeutic practice – especially Leela Anderson, Greg Smith, David Epston and Michael White.

A central principle of narrative ways of working is that the knowledges and skills of those who consult therapists shape, in significant ways, the practice of the therapy. It seems important therefore to acknowledge the significant contribution to the ideas contained in this book that has been made by those who have consulted the therapists whose work is described here.

A note about examples

In order to introduce people to narrative practices, examples of therapeutic conversations, letters and stories have been included in the following pages. These examples have been generated in a number of different ways. Some are representations of actual therapeutic conversations which all people involved are happy to see published. Others have been adapted to preserve identity by combining the elements of different people's stories. In some circumstances, in order to illustrate a specific point or way of working, a fictitious example has been used.

Please also note that in this book examples of narrative practice have been drawn from fairly traditional therapeutic settings, rather than from community contexts or from specific institutions (schools, prisons, hospitals etc.). If you'd like to read more about the use of narrative practices in these different settings please refer to the reading lists that are included throughout this book.

Part One

What is narrative therapy?

Introduction

Hello! Welcome to this easy-to-read book which is designed as an introduction to some of the main themes of narrative therapy. It includes simple and concise explanations of the thinking behind narrative practices as well as many practical examples of therapeutic conversations. This book certainly doesn't cover everything but hopefully it will serve as a starting point for further explorations. To assist this, included at the end of most of the chapters are references for further reading on various topics.

There are many different themes which make up what has come to be known as 'narrative therapy' and every therapist engages with these ideas somewhat differently. When you hear someone refer to 'narrative therapy' they might be referring to particular ways of understanding people's identities. Alternatively, they might be referring to certain ways of understanding problems and their effects on people's lives. They might also be speaking about particular ways of talking with people about their lives and problems they may be experiencing, or particular ways of understanding therapeutic relationships and the ethics or politics of therapy.

Narrative therapy seeks to be a respectful, non-blaming approach to counselling and community work, which centres people as the experts in their own lives. It views problems as separate from people and assumes people have many skills, competencies, beliefs, values, commitments and abilities that will assist them to reduce the influence of problems in their lives.

There are various principles which inform narrative ways of working, but in my opinion, two are particularly significant: always maintaining a stance of curiosity, and always asking questions to which you genuinely do not know the answers. I invite you to read this book with these two principles in mind. They inform the ideas, the stance, the tone, the values, the commitments and the beliefs of narrative therapy.

Possibilities for conversations

I have written this book in sections, each chapter describing one aspect or theme of narrative ways of working. I have done so in the hope that this

makes each element easy to understand. Instead of approaching the ideas conveyed in this book like a recipe, however, one that must be followed in a particular order, I'd invite you to instead approach them as you would a smorgasbord – an array of delicacies to choose from! I hope this book simply outlines a range of possibilities for narrative conversations.

When I meet with the people consulting me, I sometimes think of the possibilities for the directions of the conversation as if they are roads on a journey. There are many cross-roads, intersections, paths and tracks to choose from. With every step, a new and different cross road or intersection emerges – forwards, back, right, left, diagonal, in differing degrees. With each step that I take with the person consulting me, we are opening more possible directions. We can choose where to go and what to leave behind. We can always take a different path, retrace our steps, go back, repeat a track, or stay on the same road for some time. At the beginning of the journey we are not sure where it will end, nor what will be discovered.

The possibilities described in this book are like the roads, tracks and paths of the journey. Each question a narrative therapist asks is a step in a journey. All the paths may be taken, some of the paths, or one can travel along one path for a time before changing to another. There is no 'right' way to go – merely many possible directions to choose from.

Collaboration

Importantly, the person consulting the therapist plays a significant part in mapping the direction of the journey. Narrative conversations are interactive and always in collaboration with the people consulting the therapist. The therapist seeks to understand what is of interest to the people consulting them and how the journey is suiting their preferences. You will often hear, for example, a narrative therapist asking:

- *How is this conversation going for you?*

- *Should we keep talking about this or would you be more interested in ...?*

- *Is this interesting to you? Is this what we should spend our time talking about?*

- *I was wondering if you would be more interested in me asking you some more about this or whether we should focus on X, Y or Z?* [X, Y, Z being other options]

In this way, narrative conversations are guided and directed by the interests of those who are consulting the therapist.

Summary

So, before we dive into this exploration of narrative ways of working, let's quickly summarise what we have considered so far:

❖ Narrative therapy seeks to be a respectful, non-blaming approach to counselling and community work, which centres people as the experts in their own lives.

❖ It views problems as separate from people and assumes people have many skills, competencies, beliefs, values, commitments and abilities that will assist them to change their relationship with problems in their lives.

❖ Curiosity and a willingness to ask questions to which we genuinely don't know the answers are important principles of this work.

❖ There are many possible directions that any conversation can take (there is no single correct direction).

❖ The person consulting the therapist plays a significant part in determining the directions that are taken.

It seems appropriate to begin any exploration of narrative therapy with a consideration of what is meant by the 'narratives' or 'stories' of our lives.

Chapter 1

Understanding and living
our lives through stories

Narrative therapy is sometimes known as involving 're-authoring' or 're-storying' conversations. As these descriptions suggest, stories are central to an understanding of narrative ways of working.

The word 'story' has different associations and understandings for different people. For narrative therapists, stories consist of:

- events

- linked in sequence

- across time

- according to a plot

As humans, we are interpreting beings. We all have daily experiences of events that we seek to make meaningful. The stories we have about our lives are created through linking certain events together in a particular sequence across a time period, and finding a way of explaining or making sense of them. This meaning forms the plot of the story. We give meanings to our experiences constantly as we live our lives. A narrative is like a thread that weaves the events together, forming a story.

We all have many stories about our lives and relationships, occurring simultaneously. For example, we have stories about ourselves, our abilities, our struggles, our competencies, our actions, our desires, our relationships, our work, our interests, our conquests, our achievements, our failures. The way we

have developed these stories is determined by how we have linked certain events together in a sequence and by the meaning we have attributed to them.

An example: the story of my driving

I could have a story about myself as a 'good driver'. This means I could string together a number of events that have happened to me whilst driving my car. I could put these events together with others into a particular sequence and interpret them as a demonstration of me being a good driver. I might think about, and select out for the telling of the story, events such as stopping at the traffic lights, giving way to pedestrians, obeying the speed limits, incurring no fines and keeping a safe distance behind other vehicles. To form this story about my ability as a driver, I am selecting out certain events as important that fit with this particular plot. In doing so, these events are privileged over others.

As more and more events are selected and gathered into the dominant plot, the story gains richness and thickness. As it gains thickness, other events of my driving competence are easily remembered and added to the story. Throughout this process, the story thickens, becomes more dominant in my life and it is increasingly easy for me to find more examples of events that fit with the meaning I have reached.

These events of driving competence that I am remembering and selecting out are elevated in their significance over other events that do not fit with the plot of being a good driver. For instance, the times when I pulled out too quickly from the curb or misjudged the distances when parking my car are not being privileged. They might be seen as insignificant or maybe a fluke in the light of the dominant plot (a story of driving competence). In the retelling of stories, there are always events that are not selected, based upon whether or not they fit with the dominant plots.

The diagram on the next page (see figure 1) demonstrates the idea of stories consisting of events linked in sequence across time according to plot. The X marks are all the events that have occurred in my life as a driver. The events that fit with the story of 'driving competence' are scattered amongst events that are outside of that story (e.g. a car accident that occurred 4 months ago). In order to author a story of driving competence, certain events are

Figure 1

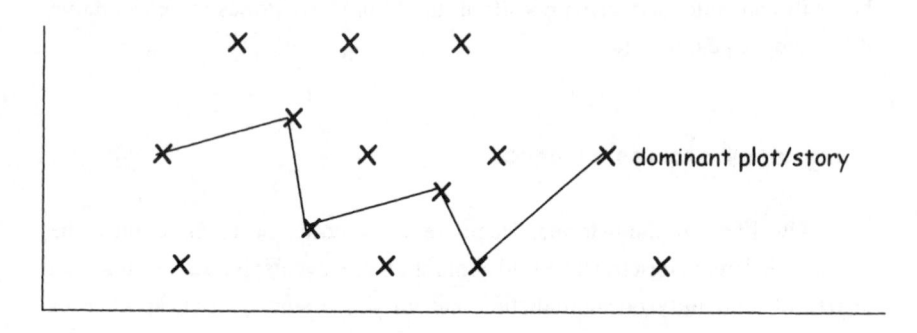

selected out and privileged over other events. Once privileged, they are linked with other events, and then still more events across time, to form a story about being a good driver. The line on the diagram shows this linking of events to form the dominant story. As you can see there are other events (X) that are outside of this dominant story that remain hidden or less significant in the light of the dominant plot.

In this example, perhaps why I can attend only to the good events, and have managed to construct a story of being a competent driver, is due to the reflections of others. If my family members and friends have always described me as a good driver, this would have made a significant difference. Stories are never produced in isolation from the broader world. Perhaps, in this example, I was never subjected to diminishing remarks on the basis of my gender. Who knows?

The effects of dominant stories

The dominant story of my driving abilities will not only affect me in the present but will also have implications for my future actions. For example, if I am asked to drive to a new suburb or drive a long distance at night, my decision and plans will be influenced by the dominant story I have about my driving. I would probably be more inclined to consider doing these things when influenced by the story I have about myself as being a good driver than if I had a story about myself as being a dangerous or accident-prone driver. Therefore,

the meanings I give to these events are not neutral in their effects on my life – they will constitute and shape my life in the future. All stories are constitutive of life and shape our lives.

Living many stories at once

Our lives are multistoried. There are many stories occurring at the same time and different stories can be told about the same events. No single story can be free of ambiguity or contradiction and no single story can encapsulate or handle all the contingencies of life.

If I had a car accident, or if someone in my life began to focus on every little mistake that I ever made while driving, or if a new law was introduced that discriminated against people like me in some way, an alternative story about my driving might begin to develop. Other events, other people's interpretations of these events, and my own interpretations could lead to an alternative story developing about my driving – a story of incompetence or carelessness. This alternative story would have effects too. For a time I might live with differing stories about my driving depending upon the context or the audience. Over time, depending on a variety of factors, the negative story about my driving might gain in influence and even become the dominant story in my life in relation to my driving. Neither the story of my driving ability nor the story of my driving failure would be free of ambiguity or contradiction.

Different types of stories

There are many different sorts of stories by which we live our lives and relationships – including stories about the past, present and future. Stories can also belong to individuals and/or communities. There can be family stories and relationship stories.

An individual may have a story about themselves as being successful and competent. Alternatively they may have a story about themselves as being 'a failure at trying new things' or 'a coward' or as 'lacking determination'. Families may have stories about themselves as being 'caring' or 'noisy' or

'risky' or 'dysfunctional' or 'close'. A community may have a story about itself as 'isolated' or 'politically active' or 'financially strong'. All these stories could be occurring at the same time, and events, as they occur, will be interpreted according to the meaning (plot) that is dominant at that time. In this way, the act of living requires that we are engaged in the mediation between the dominant stories and the alternative stories of our lives. We are always negotiating and interpreting our experiences.

The broader social context of the stories by which we live our lives

The ways in which we understand our lives are influenced by the broader stories of the culture in which we live. Some of the stories we have about our lives will have positive effects and some will have negative effects on life in the past, present and future. Laura may describe herself as a skilled therapist. She has developed this story about herself from her experiences and feedback from her work. All these experiences have contributed to shaping a story about herself as a competent, caring and skilful therapist. When faced with the decision to apply for a new job in a field that is less familiar to her, Laura is more likely to apply or think about applying under the influence of this positive self-narrative. I suspect that she would experience the challenges in her work with some confidence and might talk about her work in ways that describe it as enriching.

The meanings that we give to these events occurring in a sequence across time do not occur in a vacuum. There is always a context in which the stories of our lives are formed. This context contributes to the interpretations and meanings that we give to events. The context of gender, class, race, culture and sexual preference are powerful contributors to the plot of the stories by which we live. Laura's story of herself as a skilled therapist, for instance, would have been influenced by the ideas of the culture in which she lives. This culture would have particular beliefs about what constitutes 'skills' as a therapist and Laura's story would be shaped by these beliefs.

Laura's working-class background may have significantly contributed to the ways in which she finds it easy to make connections with people who come

to consult with her from a diversity of backgrounds. Her confidence in speaking out in work situations may have much to do with her history within the feminist movement and also the fact that as she is a white Australian professional, it is likely that people will listen to what she is saying.

In these sorts of ways, the beliefs, ideas and practices of the culture in which we live play a large part in the meanings we make of our lives.

Summary

As I have tried to explain, narrative therapists think in terms of stories – dominant stories and alternative stories; dominant plots and alternative plots; events being linked together over time that have implications for past, present and future actions; stories that are powerfully shaping of lives. Narrative therapists are interested in joining with people to explore the stories they have about their lives and relationships, their effects, their meanings and the context in which they have been formed and authored.

Chapter 2

Stories in the
therapeutic context

Let us think about some of the stories that are brought into the context of therapy. Most commonly, when people decide to consult a therapist it is because they are experiencing a difficulty or problem in their lives. When meeting with a therapist, they will often begin by telling the therapist about many events in the life of the problem for which they are seeking help. Commonly they will also explain the meanings they have given to these events.

The Craxton family sought my assistance when one of the members of the family, Sean, was caught stealing. As I heard about the problem of stealing, Sean's parents explained:

> *We are really worried about Sean because he is stealing and we have tried to stop him but he just won't. He's always been a problem child from the time he was little. He didn't get much attention when he was a small boy because Anne [his mother] was ill. Since then he always gets in trouble at school. He didn't toilet train himself and is always starting fights with his brothers. Now he's stealing to get people to notice him.*

Within this story, Sean's stealing was interpreted as meaning he was 'attention seeking'. This particular meaning (or dominant plot) occurred through a gathering together of many other events in the past that fitted with this interpretation. As Sean more and more came to be seen according to this

11

story, more and more events which supported the story of 'attention seeking' began to be selected out, and the story was told and re-told. As more events were added to this plot, the story of Sean as an 'attention seeker' became stronger.

To tell this particular story, certain events from the present and past were selected out and explained to fit with the meanings that his parents had arrived at. In doing so, certain events were selected and privileged to be told, as they were interpreted to fit with the plot of 'attention seeking'. Therefore, other events (that didn't fit with Sean as seeking attention) remained untold and unrecognised. The exceptions to this story of 'attention seeking' or times that might not fit with the 'attention seeking' story became less visible. So too, the broader cultural understandings of Sean's actions become obscured – including the fact that stealing is a common act by young men of Sean's class background in his neighbourhood. All the complexities and contradictions of Sean's life had been simplified into the understanding that Sean was an 'attention seeker'.

Thin description[1]

Early in their meetings with people, therapists often hear stories, like the one above, about the problem and the meanings that have been reached about them. These meanings, reached in the face of adversity, often consist of what narrative therapists call 'thin description'.

Thin description allows little space for the complexities and contradictions of life. It allows little space for people to articulate their own particular meanings of their actions and the context within which they occurred. For example, in the story above, the description of Sean's behaviour as 'attention seeking' was a thin description. It was generated by others (as is often the case with thin descriptions) and left little room for movement.

This thin description of Sean's actions (attention seeking) obscures many other possible meanings. For all we know, the last thing Sean wanted may have been for his stealing to be given attention! Perhaps these actions had more to do with making a stand for belonging with peers, with acquiring something for his sister, with standing up to the bullying of others, or with establishing himself as

---

[1] The term 'thin description' is borrowed from the ideas of Gilbert Ryle - see Geertz 1973.

a leader in a neighbourhood where leadership for a young man means leading break and enters (robberies). A thin description of 'attention seeking' has the potential to leave Sean isolated and disconnected from his parents and his peers, whereas alternative descriptions may open other possibilities.

Often, thin descriptions of people's actions/identities are created by others – those with the power of definition in particular circumstances (e.g. parents and teachers in the lives of children, health professionals in the lives of those who consult them). But sometimes people come to understand their own actions through thin descriptions. In whatever context thin descriptions are created, they often have significant consequences.

Thin conclusions and their effects

Thin description often leads to thin conclusions about people's identities, and these have many negative effects. For example, as Sean's actions were thinly described as 'attention seeking', he quickly became seen as 'an attention seeker'. This thin conclusion about Sean as a person was having negative effects, not only in relation to Sean's experience of himself, but also on the relationships between Sean and his parents.

Thin conclusions are often expressed as a truth about the person who is struggling with the problem and their identity. The person with the problem may be understood to be 'bad', 'hopeless', or 'a troublemaker'. These thin conclusions, drawn from problem-saturated stories, disempower people as they are regularly based in terms of weaknesses, disabilities, dysfunctions or inadequacies. I can recall many of these thin conclusions that people who have consulted me have been invited into: 'It's because I'm a bad person' or 'We are a dysfunctional family'.

Sometimes these thin conclusions obscure broader relations of power. For example, if a woman has come to see herself as 'worthless' and 'deserving of punishment' after years of being subjected to abuse, these thin conclusions make invisible the injustice she has experienced. They hide the tactics of power and control to which she has been subjected, as well as her significant acts of resistance.

Once thin conclusions take hold, it becomes very easy for people to

engage in gathering evidence to support these dominant problem-saturated stories. The influence of these problematic stories can then become bigger and bigger. In the process, any times when the person has escaped the effects of the problem, any times when they have not been 'bad', 'hopeless' or 'a trouble maker' become less visible. As the problem story gets bigger and bigger it becomes more powerful and will affect future events. Thin conclusions often lead to more thin conclusions as people's skills, knowledges, abilities and competencies become hidden by the problem story.

Alternative stories

Narrative therapists, when initially faced with seemingly overwhelming thin conclusions and problem stories, are interested in conversations that seek out alternative stories – not just any alternative stories, but stories that are identified by the person seeking counselling as stories by which they would like to live their lives. The therapist is interested to seek out, and create in conversations, stories of identity that will assist people to break from the influence of the problems they are facing.

Just as various thin descriptions and conclusions can support and sustain problems, alternative stories can reduce the influence of problems and create new possibilities for living.

For Sean, for example, an exploration of the alternative stories of his life might create space for change. These would not be stories of being an attention seeker or a problem child. Instead, they might consist of stories of determination throughout his history, or stories of how he overcame troubles in earlier times in his life, or ways in which he gives attention as well as seeks it. All of these might be alternative stories of Sean's life. Or, alternative stories might be found in other realms entirely – realms of imaginary friends, histories of connectedness with his mother or father, or within special knowledges that Sean might possess through his relationship with his beloved pet dog Rusty. In any of these territories of life, through therapeutic conversations, alternative stories might be unearthed that could assist in addressing the problems Sean is currently struggling with. The ways in which therapists and those who consult with them can co-author alternative stories will be described in following chapters.

With these ideas about stories informing their work, the key question for narrative therapists becomes: how can we assist people to break from thin conclusions and to re-author new and preferred stories for their lives and relationships?

As Jill Freedman and Gene Combs describe:

Narrative therapists are interested in working with people to bring forth and thicken stories that do not support or sustain problems. As people begin to inhabit and live out the alternative stories, the results are beyond solving problems. Within the new stories, people live out new self images, new possibilities for relationships and new futures. (1996, p.16)

Towards rich and thick description

To be freed from the influence of problematic stories, it is not enough to simply re-author an alternative story. Narrative therapists are interested in finding ways in which these alternative stories can be 'richly described'. The opposite of a 'thin conclusion' is understood by narrative therapists to be a 'rich description' of lives and relationships.

Many different things can contribute to alternative stories being 'richly described' – not least of which being that they are generated by the person whose life is being talked about. Rich description involves the articulation in fine detail of the story-lines of a person's life. If you imagine reading a novel, sometimes a story is richly described – the motives of the characters, their histories, and own understandings are finely articulated. The stories of the characters' lives are interwoven with the stories of other people and events. Similarly, narrative therapists are interested in finding ways for the alternative stories of people's lives to be richly described and interwoven with the stories of others.

The ways in which alternative stories are co-authored, how they are told and to whom, are all relevant considerations for narrative therapists. In the following pages, ways to co-author conversations that engage people in the 'rich description' of their lives and relationships will be more fully explored.

Further reading

Freedman, J. & Combs, G. 1996: 'Shifting paradigms: From systems to stories.' In Freedman, J. & Combs, G., *Narrative Therapy: The social construction of preferred realities,* chapter 1. New York: Norton.

Epston, D. & White, M. 1990: 'Story, knowledge, power.' In Epston, D. & White, M., *Narrative Means to Therapeutic Ends,* chapter 1. New York: Norton.

White, M. 1997: 'The culture of professional disciplines.' In White, M., *Narratives of Therapists' Lives,* chapter 1. Adelaide: Dulwich Centre Publications.

Chapter 3

Externalising conversations:
Naming the problem

One of the first things that a narrative therapist is interested in doing is to separate the person's identity from the problem for which they seek assistance. They therefore begin speaking about the problem in ways that situate it separately from the person and their identity. This is based on the premise that the problem is the problem, as opposed to the person being seen as the problem.

Externalising conversations, which occur all the time in narrative therapy, are ways of speaking that separate problems from people. Externalisation is the foundation from which many, though by no means all, narrative conversations are built. Externalisation requires a particular shift in the use of language. It is an attitude and orientation in conversations, not simply a technique or skill. This is an important distinction to make because, if externalising is used as simply a technique, it can often have the opposite effect to that intended.

When people seek the assistance of a therapist, they often speak about the problem in ways that assume that it is somehow part of them, or within them, for example:

- *I am a depressive sort of person and don't want to go anywhere.*

- *I'm unmotivated and just can't seem to get the energy to do anything.*

- *I am a worrier. I always get anxious when I try new things.*

These internalising conversations (conversations that locate problems inwardly) usually have negative effects on people's lives and result in thin conclusions (as described in chapter 2).

A narrative therapist listens to these descriptions and is interested in engaging in a conversation to situate the problem away from the person – to externalise it. So instead of 'I'm unmotivated, I can't do anything', the therapist might say 'So the problem has affected your energy levels'. Instead of 'I am a depressive sort of person', the therapist could say 'So the Depression has made it hard for you to go out' or 'When the Problem is strong it has you thinking that you have no motivation'. 'I am a worrier' could be externalised by saying something like 'The Worry tries to stop you from trying new things'.[2]

Within externalising conversations, problems are always spoken of as separate from people. To assist therapists when first exploring externalising conversations, I sometimes suggest that they imagine the problem as being a 'thing' that is sitting somewhere else in the room, for example, on the person's shoulder, or on a different chair. Thinking about it in this way can help therapists to separate in their own minds the person from the problem.

There are many ways to begin externalising conversations. The therapist's language, choice of words and the way in which s/he phrases sentences and questions are all crucial. The phrasing of statements and questions shifts the conversation from an internalised conversation to an externalised one. (See Table 1: 'Some differences between internalising and externalising conversations' at the end of this chapter.)

Narrative therapists will listen to the description of the person's experience, hoping to hear a word or phrase that describes what might be getting in the way of the person's life. They are listening for the names or ways of referring to the problem that the person consulting them uses. A person may say 'I just get so worried that I can't sleep at night', and 'It's like a negative voice inside my head telling me that I can't do anything'. The person has used the word 'worry' and 'the negative voice' to refer to the problem so the therapist may pick up on these two words.

These words would then be used by the therapist and phrased differently so that it is clear the problem is situated outside of the person and their identity.

---

[2] When writing about a problem, therapists often give the problem's name a capital letter to assist in further externalising it.

The therapist might make a statement such as 'So the Worry is stopping you from sleeping at night', or ask a question like: 'How has the Negative Voice tried to convince you that you can't do anything?' Placing the word 'the' before the problem name immediately situates it away from the person. In externalised conversations, often an adjective or verb becomes a noun. For example, the word 'depressed' would become 'the Depression', 'fighting' would be spoken of as 'the Fighting', or 'worried' as 'the Worry'.

Sometimes the problem can be given an identity or a name like a person (this is called personifying the problem). People who consult me about the effects of anorexia nervosa on their lives sometimes choose to refer to the problem as 'Rex' or 'The demon' or 'Fred' or sometimes 'Anorexia'. Some children who have been experiencing enuresis or encopresis have chosen to call the problem 'Sneaky wee' or 'Tricky poo'. Tempers have sometimes been referred to as 'The Temper Tyrant'.

Asking people, particularly children, to draw what the problem looks like can sometimes also be helpful. Therapists often find this a useful way to help them separate the person from the problem (see below).

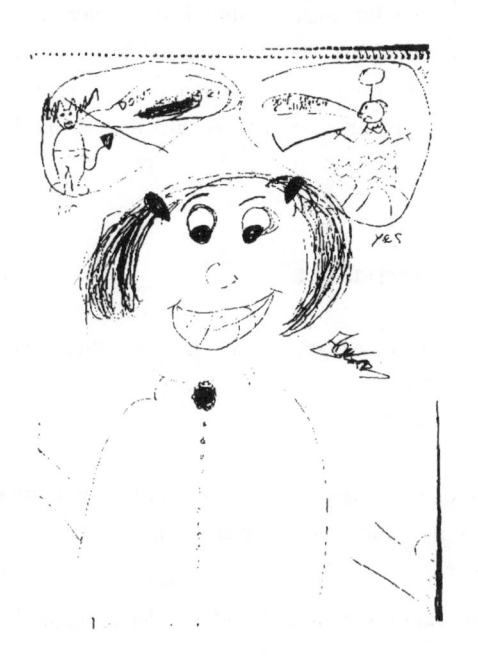

Naming the problem

Importantly, the language and name for the problem comes from the person consulting the therapist and is selected by them. The therapist may ask something like 'I'm just wondering if there is a name you would give to this problem?' and invite them to choose an appropriate name.

The therapist might hesitantly suggest a name or way of referring to the problem. 'I was wondering about what you would call this problem, something like, the Depression or the Worry or the Guilt or Self-doubt? They were some of the things I was thinking of whilst you were speaking. What do you think?' The therapist would be extremely tentative to be sure that the name is one that appeals to the person consulting them. The therapist does not want in any way to impose a name on them. They may check the words with the person by saying something like: 'I was wondering if the name Anxiety or Worry would fit for you? We could just keep calling the problem "It" until we come up with a better one, if that is easier ...'.

Initially the problem might simply be named 'It' until a name that suits the person consulting the therapist is found. During the course of a conversation or a series of therapy sessions, the name that has been agreed upon to describe the problem can change as more is discovered about its characteristics. It is very important that the therapist continually consults the person during re-authoring conversations.

What can be externalised?

In the course of conversations many different things can be externalised.

Feelings

Feelings such as anxiety, worry, fear, guilt, depression may be the focus of externalising conversations. In these situations, therapists might phrase their questions like these:

- *So what has the Guilt tried to talk you into about yourself?*

- *So how has the Fear tried to convince you that it is unsafe go out of your own house?*

- *How long has the Jealousy been trying to get between you and your friends?*

Problems between people

Aspects of interpersonal relationships may also be externalised, e.g., the Bickering, the Blame, the Criticism, the Fighting, the Hopelessness, the Mistrust, the Jealousy. Questions in these situations could sound like:

- *What have the Fights talked you into about yourself as a partner?*

- *What does the Blame have you doing with each other?*

- *What is the Conflict talking you into about each other?*

- *How much does the Bickering get in the way of your conversations?*

Cultural and social practices

Cultural and social practices may also be situated away from the person. Mother-blaming, parent-blaming, women-blaming, heterosexual dominance, racism, economic rationalism may be named as practices that have assisted the problem to increase its influence in a person's life.

Other metaphors

Sometimes people may talk about a problem metaphorically. For example, they may speak of a 'wall of resentment', 'the block', 'the dream', or 'the tidal wave of despair'. Metaphors like these can also be externalised.

More than one problem at a time

In the course of a conversation it is possible that there will be more than one problem externalised. In this situation, the therapist might name and list all of the externalised problems and ask the person consulting them to prioritise them. Alternatively, it is often possible to be flexible and open to externalising various problematic situations as they arise in the conversation. It may be that one problem is working together with another problem. Depression may have

'friends' or 'allies' that assist it. It might be teaming up with 'Self-doubt' or 'Self-criticism', for example.

Taking care to consider the broader context

Taking care when choosing words to represent the problem is very important in externalising conversations. It is crucial that the language chosen in externalising conversations does not inadvertently reinforce dominant ideas that may be supporting the problem. Some externalisations will create much more room to move than others.

For example, if I was consulting a child in relation to their experiences of bullying in the schoolyard and they spoke equally about the effects of 'Sadness' and the effects of 'Hassling', I would be interested in asking some further questions to determine what to externalise. Knowing that focusing on externalising sadness in this sort of situation could inadvertently contribute to making invisible the relations of power that were occurring in this child's life, I might ask whether it is the Hassling that brings the Sadness? Or, is Sadness around more or less when Hassling is around? If the answer did link the Sadness to Hassling then I might ask if it would be all right to ask some more questions about Hassling. In this way I would be keeping an awareness of the politics involved in naming the problem, while also consulting with the child to ensure that we came up with a name for the problem that truly represented her/his experience.

It is important that the context of a person's life is always addressed in externalising conversations. If, for example, a young person is brought to therapy with his/her family complaining of anger and tantrums, one initially might consider externalising this problem as 'the Tantrums' or 'Temper'. What if, however, the family has recently moved house because of a change in their financial circumstances? What if the young person and family were also experiencing the effects of racism? These contextual factors could be minimised if the problem was named as 'Temper', and a further injustice could be done. Taking care to explore the social context in which the problem is occurring is therefore an important part of externalising conversations. In this situation, after further conversations the problem might perhaps be named 'the Rage' in a way

that takes into account the relevant issues of power and injustice in the young person's life.

Another important factor in relation to acknowledging the broader context of people's lives in externalising conversations relates to issues of abuse. Because of the prevalence of abuse, checking out whether it is a part of the context of a person's life needs to be routine. This is particularly true in relation to children. In some circumstances, when thinking about externalising conversations, checking out about the possibility of abuse is crucial. If a child, for example, was speaking about the fear in their life, the terrors, or the nightmares they were experiencing, these would not be externalised until there was a thorough exploration of the context of the child's life. This exploration of the context of the child's life is needed in order to ensure that abuse is not the reason for the terror, fear or nightmares.[3] To name a problem as fear/terror/ nightmares when the problem is actually one of abuse could contribute to silencing the child's experience, and reduce the likelihood of the abuse being addressed. In this way, as a part of determining the course of externalising conversations, therapists need to be constantly checking out the broader context of people's lives. Externalising conversations need to be seen in the context of these checking-out processes and a constant awareness of the broader context of people's lives.

So, in summary, within externalising conversations it is important that: the name of the problem fits the experience of the person consulting the therapist; that the person consulting the therapist is actively involved in deciding upon how the problem is going to be referred to; and that the name chosen allows for the politics of experience to be examined. If therapists have any dilemmas about what to externalise they may need to ask further questions to the person(s) concerned to clarify what would be the best way to refer to the problem.

---

[3] For a further consideration of ways of working in relation to issues of abuse see Kamsler 1990, White 1995.

Why do we choose to engage in externalising conversations?

People who are engaged in externalising conversations find them extremely helpful for many reasons. Externalising conversations establish a context where the person experiences themselves as separate from the problem. In this way the problem no longer speaks to them of their identity or the 'truth' about who they are. People often find this a great relief as it opens space for them to begin to take action against the problem and opens space for them to work co-operatively to revise their relationship with the problem.

Problems appear less fixed and less restricting when spoken of in externalising ways. When people are separated from problems, their skills, abilities, interests, competencies and commitments become more visible. The more visible these skills become, the more available they are for people to access. Externalising conversations reduce guilt and blame and yet leave room for responsibility.

Externalising conversations begin to disempower the effects of labelling, pathologising and diagnosing that are commonly experienced by people as impoverishing of their lives. They open possibilities for people to describe themselves, each other and their relationships from a new and non-problem-saturated position. Externalising conversations facilitate the renaming of the problem-saturated story that once dominated their lives. In this way, 'the problem becomes the problem and then the person's relationship with the problem becomes the problem'.(White & Epston 1990, p.40) Externalising conversations enable the development of an alternative story for family life that is more attractive to family members.

Once a person is separated from the problem or the dominant problem story, once they begin speaking about themselves as being affected by the problem as opposed to themselves being problematic, options become available. Times or ways in which they have been or are presently separated from the effects of the problem become easier to think and speak about. These times are known as 'unique outcomes' and will be discussed in chapter 7. Unique outcomes provide openings to different stories and rich descriptions of people's lives.

Externalising conversations can also decrease the amount of unproductive conflict that may have arisen between people since the problem's

existence. Disputes over who is to blame become less relevant as people begin to think of the problem as an independent entity. Co-operation and collaboration become more of a possibility when the problem is not located within the identity of either person.

A thorough exploration and personification of the problem

Agreeing upon a way of referring to the problem and engaging in an externalising conversation shifts the problem from inside the person to outside of them. A thorough investigation into the problem is then possible. This thorough investigation can occur at any time in conversations with people.

The therapist is interested in exposing and finding out as much as possible about:

- the problem's tricks
- the problem's tactics
- the problem's way of operating
- the problem's ways of speaking: its voice, tone, the content of what it says
- the problem's intentions
- the problem's beliefs and ideas,
- the problem's plans
- the problem's likes and dislikes
- the problem's rules
- the problem's purposes
- the problem's desires
- the problem's motives
- the problem's techniques
- the problem's dreams
- the problem's allies: who stands with it or beside it; who supports it; what forces are in league with it
- the problem's deceits or lies

As we discuss all these facets the problem gradually develops its own persona. Exploring widely the problem's tricks and methods of operation, and doing this in some detail, identifies the problem as a separate 'thing' or being. This is why these sorts of conversations are sometimes referred to as conversations which 'personify the problem'. The questions that are asked lead to the problem being identified as having its own ways of living and its own motives, distinct from those of the person seeking assistance.

One way to explain this type of conversation is to introduce you to Madeline, who was eight years old when we met. Madeline consulted me about the effects of 'the Dumb Bug' in her life. The Dumb Bug was getting in the way of her concentration at school and making it hard for Madeline to try new things. During our initial meetings together I asked Madeline a lot of questions about the Dumb Bug and what it was up to. I will summarise some of the things that Madeline told me and the questions I asked her. They are drawn from a number of conversations over a period of time.

Alice: So what does the Dumb Bug tell you about yourself?

Madeline: It says I can't do anything and tries to stop me from trying.

Alice: How does it stop you from trying?

Madeline: It says, 'You won't be able to do that. It's too hard. There's no point even starting, 'cos you won't be able to do it'.

Alice: How does it say that? Does it have a special sort of voice or way of speaking?

Madeline: Oh … it's sort of a loud voice.

Alice: A loud voice?

Madeline: It booms at me and yells at me and says it meanly.

Alice: Does it always speak meanly to you?

Madeline: Always. It never says anything nice, just things like 'You are dumb', 'You are stupid'.

Alice: When does it say these things? Is it all the time or only some of the time?

Madeline: Just some of the time but usually when I get my work from the teacher and also it says things to me at sport.

Alice: What does it say at sport?

Madeline: 'You're dumb, you can't play in that team because the other kids won't want you.'

Alice: So it criticises you? Is that right?

Madeline: Yes, it always criticises me, in everything; even when I am at home it criticises how I dry the dishes.

Alice: How does the Dumb Bug work? Do you know it's coming? Does it give you any warnings?

Madeline: Sometimes I know it's there because it makes my stomach churn.

Alice: So it targets your stomach first? Is that right?

Madeline: No. Before that it is in my head saying things and then it goes to my stomach.

Alice: Then what happens?

Madeline: Well then it has got me because when my stomach churns, I can't do anything and I can't think.

Alice: So its tactic is to first grab your thoughts and then it works on your stomach.

Madeline: Yes

Alice: How long would it take to do this? Does it work quickly or slowly?

Madeline: Once it puts its mind to it, the Dumb Bug moves fast.

All problems can be externalised. Fear, anxiety, anorexia nervosa, voices of schizophrenia, racism, habits, illness, self-doubt, all have particular methods of operation. There can be similarities between the way in which problems speak and there can be differences.

For example, many women have told me that the voice of anorexia nervosa is a male voice. However, some say it speaks in a soft and subtle voice, whilst others say that it speaks in a bossy and booming voice. They all say that it tells them they will get fat if they eat. To some women Anorexia Nervosa speaks to them all the time, to others it speaks only at meal times and when they see food.

Therapists never presume they 'know' how the problem works. Each conversation is treated as separate from all others. Sometimes the therapist's experience with other people can be drawn upon to assist with the expose of the problem. I could, for example, say to Madeline: 'I've spoken to a few people now who have had some experience with something like the Dumb Bug. Would you be interested in knowing what they have said about that? They have said that the Dumb Bug likes them to give up easily and not try anything. Has it tried that on you or does it try different things?' Madeline's response to this question will open more possibilities to explore how the Dumb Bug operates.

It is helpful to explore carefully all aspects of the problem as this can further assist the person to separate themselves from it. This exploration may occur at any time – from the first minutes of the conversation. Throughout the conversations, it is up to the therapist to listen for signs of the tactics of the problem. Once the problem has been externalised, if the therapist ever suspects that the problem's tactics are present in the conversation (if the problem is affecting the ways in which the person is speaking) then the therapist may choose to investigate this by asking a series of questions. They may also initiate an exploration of the tactics of the problem and its effects and consult the person about their interest in pursuing this sort of direction for their life and relationships.

Revising relationships with problems

By enabling people to separate themselves from the problems about which they are seeking assistance, externalising conversations allow for explorations of the relationship *between* the person and the problem. When we keep in mind that people are in a particular relationship with the problem for which they seek help, this opens possibilities for re-authoring conversations.

Therapists can ask people to think of ways to describe the relationship that currently exists between them and the problem. Questions may sound something like this: 'Is there a name you could give to how things are between you and Perfectionism?' or 'What words would you use to describe your relationship with this problem? Is it a happy relationship, or a sad one or a mixed type of connection?' People may use words like 'troubled',

'argumentative', 'conflictual', 'love/hate', 'friendly' or 'friend and foe'. Sometimes metaphors may be evoked such as 'It's like a saga' or 'It's like being ruled by a tyrant'. These explorations can assist in describing the nature of the relationship between the person and the problem.

Once a description has been given to the current relationship, the therapist might ask some questions to determine what type of relationship would better suit the person. This allows people to begin to state their own opinions and ideas and can be an important step in the process of re-authoring lives. It might be that people wish to end their relationship with the problem. In other situations people might simply be hoping for a 'calm', 'occasional' or 'trouble-free' relationship with what is currently a problem.

The following chapters will explore ways in which therapeutic conversations can assist people to change the relationships they have with problems. First, however, I have included a table that maps out some of the differences between internalising and externalising conversations.

Table 1: Some differences between internalised and externalised conversations

Internalised conversations	*Externalised conversations*
See the person as the problem.	See the problem as the problem.
Locate problems inside the person.	The problem is spoken of as outside of the person. This creates space for discussion about the person's relationship with the problem.
Look for what is 'wrong' or 'deficient' with individuals.	Locate problems in a context that is external or outside of the person and their identity.
Actions seen as surface manifestations of a central core or self.	Actions seen as events that have occurred in a sequence, across a time period according to a particular plot.

Internalised conversations (cont'd)	*Externalised conversations* (cont'd)
Seek the opinions of others to explain behaviours or problems.	Invite people to discern their own meaning and explanations for events.
Descriptions tend to totalise the person and their identity leaving little room for other descriptions of identity.	Allow for multiple descriptions of identity.
Make invisible the social practices that promote, sustain and nurture the life of the problem.	Make visible the social practices that promote, sustain and nurture the life of the problem.
Lead to thin conclusions about life, the self, and relationships.	Lead to rich descriptions of lives and relationships.
Examine the internal influences on people who seek help.	Examine the cultural, socio-political stories that influence the lives of people who seek help.
Lead to categorisation of people in terms of how 'different' they are from the 'norm'. Labels or terms are devised to describe people's experience or problem. When people are seen as different, they often experience discrimination.	Celebrate difference and challenge notions of 'norms'. Embrace difference and seek to make discriminatory practices visible.
Understand problems as 'part of people and their identity'. Conversations are therefore centred around ways of 'living with' the effects of certain diagnoses, e.g. 'autism' or 'ADD'.	Involve consulting people about changing or re-negotiating relationships with problems.

Those outside of the influence of the problem (e.g. professionals) are seen as the experts.	People hold the expertise over their own lives and relationships.
The agent of change is considered to be the strategies designed by others that will 'fix' the problem.	The agent of change is communal. Externalising conversations seek to discover what skills and knowledges are present.
Language used is often 'I am ...'	Language used is often 'It is ...'
Often involve talking a lot about the problem and its details.	Seek alternative descriptions and stories outside of the problem description.

Further reading

Morgan, A. 1998: 'Conversations of ability.' In White, C. & Denborough, D. (eds), *Introducing Narrative Therapy: A collection of practice based writing.* Adelaide: Dulwich Centre Publications

White, M. & Epston, D. 1990: 'Externalising of the problem.' In White, M. & Epston, D. (co-authors), *Narrative Means to Therapeutic Ends,* chapter 2, pp.38-76. New York: Norton.

For examples of externalising conversations in community work settings see:

The work of the CARE Counsellors of Malawi & Sliep, Y. 1998: 'Pang'ono pang'ono ndi mtolo – little by little we make a bundle.' In White, C. & Denborough, D. (eds), *Introducing Narrative Therapy: A collection of practice based-writings.* Adelaide: Dulwich Centre Publications.

Wingard, B. 1998: 'Introducing "sugar".' In White, C. & Denborough, D. (eds), *Introducing Narrative Therapy: A collection of practice-based writings.* Adelaide: Dulwich Centre Publications.

Wingard, B. 1998: 'Grief: Remember, reflect, reveal.' In White, C. & Denborough, D. (eds), *Introducing Narrative Therapy: A collection of practice-based writings.* Adelaide: Dulwich Centre Publications.

Chapter 4

Tracing the history
of the problem

Early in their meetings with people, therapists interested in narrative practices often facilitate externalising conversations with the person consulting them (as discussed in the previous chapter). Once a conversation is opened whereby the problem is named and separated from the person, the therapist is interested in asking some questions that inquire into the history of the problem in the person's life. This history may include anything from the distant past (perhaps before the problem entered the person's life) through to the nearer past (perhaps the day before, the minute before, the previous week, the time since making the appointment). This inquiry tries to trace the influence of the problem in the person's life over a long time period.

Often this inquiry will come from things that the person consulting the therapist says, such as: 'It is funny, you know, because when I was on holidays last year I really felt different and the illness didn't get in the way at all' or 'I don't even remember having self-doubt as a child'. The therapist may pick up on statements such as these and inquire further by asking for more details about the times referred to and the times after and before it, for example: 'How old were you then when you were free from self-doubt?' and 'Since that time can you fill me in on what it has been like?'

The therapist can also ask more direct questions about the past and the person's relationship with the problem at those times. The therapist is seeking to

understand events in the past and what the person noticed about the problem at that time. Some questions might include:

- *When did you first notice the problem? How long ago?*

- *What do you remember before the problem entered your life?*

- *When would you say the problem was strongest? When was it weakest? When did you feel stronger in the face of the problem?*

- *What was it like for you 6 months ago [3 months ago, 1 year ago, 4 years ago, 3 days ago]? What did you notice about the problem? How much of your life did it have at that time?*

In these questions, the therapist may simply refer to the problem as 'the problem' or use the particular externalised name or metaphor that has been negotiated, for example: 'When would you say that Self-Doubt was strongest?' Specifying the problem's name in this externalised way further assists to separate the problem from the person.

The therapist can choose any time frame in order to explore the life of the person and the life of the problem. Questions that begin with What, Where, When and Who can facilitate conversations that provide more specific details about the events at that time.

Relative influence questioning

Relative influence questions can be helpful when tracing the history of the problem. The therapist can ask the person to imagine they were to think about their life as a total of the number ten. The therapist can then ask: 'How much of your life out of ten would you say the problem had six months ago and how much of your life did you have?' The person may reply, 'Six months ago It had six out of ten and I had four out of ten'. The therapist can then ask about other time periods using the same numerical system: 'And a week ago, what would you say you had and how much did the problem have?' The person may say, 'Oh, eight out of ten to the problem and two out of ten to me'.

These questions allow the therapist to inquire about any time during the past. There are many sorts of relative influence questions that can be used.

Questions can be asked that invite the person to consider the influence of the problem with numbers: e.g. out of 10, 20, 50, 100, or as a percentage. Or people might be interested in drawing a pictorial representation.

Amy found it helpful to draw a line and divide it into segments to show the influence of worry in her life. The complete line represents Amy's life. I asked Amy to mark an X to show how much of her life worry had and how much she had at different points in time.

**The part of Amy's life
taken up with Worry**
                                    **The part of Amy's life
separate from Worry**

Yesterday:
_____X_____

Three weeks ago:
_____X_____

Two months ago:
_____X_____

One year ago:
_____X_____

Four years ago:
_____X_____

Five years ago:
_____X_____

From these pictures we began to get a view of Amy's life and the problem's life.

Allyssa chose to represent her life by drawing a spiral shape. She marked on the spiral the amount of space she had and the amount of space the problem had at different times in her life.

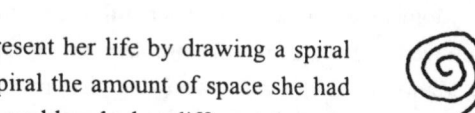

Elenni did this by drawing a picture to represent the size of herself and the size of the problem at particular times. She explained to me that there are times when she is bigger than Trouble and times when Trouble is bigger than her.

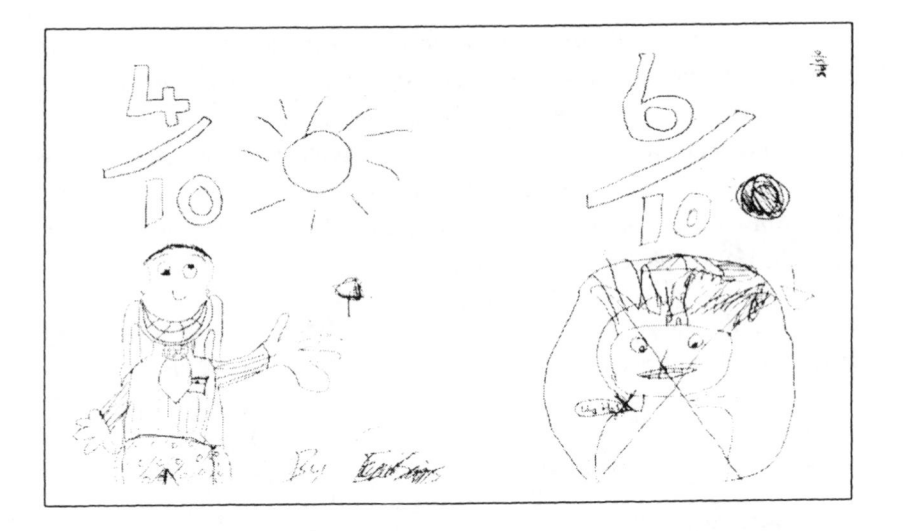

Fractions are another way to show the problem's influence over time. The therapist can ask the person for example to shade in a shape (square, circle, triangle, a blob shape) to depict the amount of problem's life and the amount of their life over time. Some therapists might ask a person to cut a piece of paper into two pieces; one piece to represent the size of the problem and one to represent the size of the person's life.

Why is it helpful?

Tracing the history of the problem in the person's life begins to open space for the consideration of other stories about the problem. When the problem is placed in a context over time, it is seen as changing and less static or fixed. Moments of greater or lesser influence can be identified. People often feel relieved to discover that the problem has changed at different times in their lives. Manisha said to me: 'Knowing that makes my future seem brighter because I can see that I'm not stuck with this. The problem doesn't seem as huge now.'

When times of lesser and greater influence are discovered, new or different stories may emerge. Times when the problem had less influence (or perhaps no influence) may be unique outcomes (see chapter 7) and lead to an

exploration of the person's skills and competencies at that time.

Conversations that trace the history of the problem enable the therapist to get a sense of some of the meanings (thin conclusions) that the person may have reached during the problem's existence. For example, Tony said, 'The anxiety was really strong before coming here because I don't cope well with new situations'. These thin conclusions can then be explored further in conversations in ways that open up possibilities for new and different meanings.

Tracing the history of the problem can also make it possible to discover how the person has been influential over the problem at particular times. The therapist may ask about the times when for instance they had 8 out of 10 of their life and the problem only had 2. The therapist may seek to understand more about what was happening at that time, the skills, competencies, desires or hopes the person was connected to and the ways they were reducing the influence of the problem at that time. This can open very different non-problem-saturated conversations.

Asking questions that trace the problem's history may also begin to identify some of the problem's tactics and methods of operation (see chapter 3 Personifying the problem). For example, when Tony told his therapist that anxiety likes to have him feel worried about new situations and that anxiety had tried to stop him from coming to the therapy appointment, the therapist might have been interested in asking more about how anxiety works. This might have led into an exploration of other times when anxiety had tried to prevent him taking some sort of action but had failed.

Externalising conversations that trace the history of the problem over time contribute to the person further separating from the problem as they place the problem in a longer term context. As soon as these conversations are taking place, re-storying work has begun.

Problems that seem to have a long history

Considerations of history are also important when discussing problems that have been around for a long time. Tracing the history of these sorts of problems enables long-term problems to be placed within a storyline. Questions can be asked that lead to an exploration of when the problem first came into a

person's life, when the problem story took shape, how it was supported and who it was supported by. A sense of history enables the problem to be placed within a plot or a storyline.

For example, Raul was suffering from severe depression. For much of his adult life he had lived alone with little interaction with others. Depression had accompanied him since he was a young man. He had been hospitalised on a number of occasions, and was consulting a therapist now because he was concerned that he wished to end his life. In the course of conversations, the history of Depression entering his life was gradually articulated. In time, Raul could identify the very day it had first appeared in his life. This was the day his mother had died and he was sent to live in a foster home that would prove to be an abusive and hostile place. By tracing Depression's entry into his life at this moment, Raul was able to speak about his life before Depression, his life with his mother and the loving times they had shared together. He was able to trace the tactics of Depression and the abuse that had enabled it to claim most of his life. Over time, placing Depression into a plot, or storyline also enabled Raul to consider the histories of the ways in which he had tried to resist Depression's influence. By finding ways to acknowledge these histories, and finding ways to reconnect with his mother's image, Depression's influence ever so gradually began to have less of a hold on Raul's life.

I shall write more about tracing the histories of resistance to problems in chapter 8. But prior to exploring the ways in which people have resisted problems, it is important for the effects of the problem to be fully explored.

Further reading

White, M. 1993: 'Histories of the present.' In Gilligan, S. (ed), *Therapeutic Conversations.* New York: Norton.

Chapter 5

Exploring the effects
of the problem

Early on in therapeutic conversations, it is important to explore in some detail the effects that the problem has had on the person's life. Again, the problem is spoken of as external to the person's identity (see chapter 3). The therapist can ask a series of questions about the ways in which the problem has affected:

- the person's sense of self: what they think of themselves as a person
- their view of themselves as a parent, partner, mother, wife, sister, brother, worker, etc.
- their hopes, dreams and sense of the future
- their relationships with children, parents, partner, community members, colleagues, etc.
- their work
- their social life
- their thoughts
- their physical health
- their spirits
- their moods or feelings
- their everyday life

The questions might sound something like these:

- *How have the Habits affected your relationship with your teacher? Has it got you closer or further from him?*

- *How has the Depression affected how you think about yourself?*

- *How have the Hostile Voices affected your energy levels? Is it easier or harder to do things when they are dominant?*

- *How has the Bulimia affected your moods and feelings?*

- *How has the Fear affected your beliefs about other people and the wider world?*

- *Have the Tantrums affected your work?*

- *What effect has the Worry had on your view of yourself as a father?*

- *What effect has the Fighting had on your social life? Have you noticed any changes?*

- *How has the Injury affected how you see yourself as a parent and partner?*

Why is this helpful?

It is important to map these effects widely and spend time exploring them carefully so that an understanding of the impact of the dominant problem story in the person's life is fully appreciated. These conversations act as a powerful acknowledgement of the distress and/or worry that the person consulting the therapist may be experiencing. Without these explorations of the effects of the problem on the person's life, it can feel as if the therapist has not really understood or listened to the experience of the person seeking consultation. When more than one person is present at a meeting, each family member can be consulted about the effects of the problem on their own life. This may bring to light similarities and differences in experience that can then be further explored.

Therapists may use written documents (see chapter 10) to powerfully acknowledge the effects that the problem is having on the person's life. The

more particular the exploration of effects of the problem, the more effective it can be. It is important to note that this exploration of the effects needs to occur only through externalising conversations, for example, 'So the hostile voices have you feeling worthless?' If these explorations did not occur in externalising ways, they could quite easily contribute to the person feeling worse as the problem's influence could inadvertently be increased. If the tracing of the effects happens in externalising ways, however, it can be an empowering, clarifying and acknowledging process. It can reduce the sense of isolation that the problem may have been causing and it can be a sane-making process by clarifying that there are reasons why the person is feeling as burdened as they are – that these are the effects of the problem.

Exploring in detail the effects of the problem may also lead to the discovery of unique outcomes – times in the life of the person when the problem has not been influential (see chapter 7). It is important that therapists are constantly oriented towards listening for these times.

Rosy consulted me about the effects of anorexia nervosa on her life. When I asked her about the effects anorexia was having on her moods, Rosy told me that she often felt really 'touchy, moody and tired' since anorexia had entered her life. She had also noticed that it was more difficult to concentrate and that anorexia had isolated her from her friends and family. As I inquired about the effect of anorexia on her work, Rosy told me: 'Oh no, it doesn't get in the way of work. No-one has noticed anything. I try really hard not to let it get in the way of work. My work is really important to me.' This was significant to Rosy and led to a conversation that explored how Rosy was able to do this. This opened a new and different story concerning Rosy and her relationship with anorexia nervosa.

Questions that explore the effects of the problem allow for an alternative story to emerge. They help to open the possibility of noticing ways that people are coping or managing in the face of the problem, to highlight the abilities and competencies they are drawing on to assist them.

It is important that therapists do not move too quickly to explore these different times or unique outcomes (see chapter 7). If a person has chosen to come to a therapist, the chances are that the problem-story is quite influential and has been having significant effects on the person's life. It is important the therapist explores these effects, and in this way acknowledges them.

These sorts of conversations are also helpful in exposing some of the tactics and tricks that problems use against people. Very often, it is in a problem's interest to try to disguise their effects on people – problems do not like people to notice what they are up to! The act of speaking about the effects of problems is often against the problem's interests and has the potential to reduce the problem's influence in and of itself. By exposing the tactics and effects of the problem, these conversations strengthen the person's voice and opinions.

Evaluating the effects of the problem

As the effects of the problem are fully explored, the therapist asks the person to consider each effect and asks their opinion on them. The therapist is interested in understanding how each effect suits or does not suit the person's life. There are a number of ways the therapist might do this.

Questions might include:

- *What is that like for you and your family?*
- *Is that a good thing or a bad thing?*
- *Does this please you or not?*
- *What is your experience of that – positive or negative?*
- *Is that something you would like more of or less of?*
- *Is this a positive or negative development?*
- *How does this suit you?*

The person is given time to state their position on each effect. This is important because the therapist does not presume anything about the person's experience of the problem. When I asked Rosy about the effects of anorexia nervosa that she had described to me, she thought that being tired and moody was something she would like less of, and that it did not suit her for anorexia to be interfering with her friendships. Rosy also thought it was a good thing that anorexia did not affect her working life and wanted this to continue.

The therapist can never know what the effects of the problem mean to the person whose life they are discussing. Only the person themselves knows

this and the therapist needs to consult them in order to ensure that they understand the situation.

Justification of the evaluation

As the therapist inquires as to the position that the person takes on the effects of the problem on their lives, they then ask the simple question 'Why?' This question is very important as it seeks to elicit a justification as to why they evaluate the effects of problem in a certain way. This process often draws attention to many aspects of the person's preferences for living. When I asked Rosy why it did not suit her to be tired and moody, she said 'Because I used to be such a happy person and nice to be around and people liked to be with me'. She also said that she did not like anorexia interfering with her friendships because 'I have had those friends for a long time now and they are very special to me. I enjoy their company and we used to have lots of fun together.' Rosy explained that it was good that anorexia was not affecting her work because 'I love my work and it is important to me, and something I'm really interested in'.

From these justifications it is possible to begin to develop a different story about Rosy and her interests, ideas, beliefs, skills, preferences and ideas. These opinions of Rosy and her hopes for her life were potentially being overshadowed by the dominant story of anorexia. Drawing attention to these opinions and hopes can assist a process of reconnection with them. Creating a context for people to reconnect with their preferences and opinions can be a significant part of re-authoring conversations.

Through these conversations the person is invited to take a position in relation to the problem. This assists people to shift from the problem-saturated story into a new territory of their life that is consistent with *their* values, skills, competencies and preferences for living. As will be discussed further in chapter 7, unique outcomes emerge when people are asked to justify the effects of the problem on their lives and relationships. These conversations help people to be clearer on where they stand in relation to the problem and this in itself can contribute to a reduction of the influence of the problem and the creation of alternative stories.

Summary

The steps outlined in the last two sections are referred to by Michael White as 'The statement of position map'. To summarise:

❖ Naming the problem – negotiating a definition of the problem that fits with the meaning and experience of the person whose life the problem is affecting.

❖ Effects – exploring the effects of the problem.

❖ Evaluate – inviting the person to evaluate these effects.

❖ Justify – inviting the person to justify their evaluation: Why?

Chapter 6

Situating the problem in context:
Deconstruction

From a narrative therapy perspective, problems only survive and thrive when they are supported and backed up by particular ideas, beliefs and principles. Acts of men's violence and abuse against women, for example, can only exist when they are supported by ideas of patriarchy and male dominance that serve to justify and excuse this violence. Anorexia and bulimia nervosa can only survive in cultures that value thinness, where success and competence are judged in terms of body shape and size, and in cultures which promote self-surveillance and individualism.

Narrative therapists are interested in discovering, acknowledging and 'taking apart' (deconstructing) the beliefs, ideas and practices of the broader culture in which a person lives that are serving to assist the problem and the problem story. In this way, the cultural beliefs that have assisted the problem to come into the person's life, and the beliefs and ideas that are assisting in sustaining the life of the problem, become more available for questioning and challenge. The beliefs and ideas that are assisting problems are often regarded as 'taken for granted', as 'truths', or as 'common-place understandings'. Through questions and conversation, therapists can work with the people consulting them to examine these ideas and practices, define them, pull them

apart and trace their history.

Throughout their meetings with people, therapists can consider the context in which the problem story exists, the ideas and beliefs that are sustaining the problem and the history of the ideas. They listen for and ask themselves:

- *What are the background assumptions that enable this story to make sense?*

- *What unnamed background assumptions make this story work?*

- *What are the ideas that might explain how people are speaking and acting?*

- *What are some of the taken-for-granted ways of living and being that are assisting the life of the problem?*

The pulling apart and examining of 'taken-for-granted' truths is known as deconstruction. Deconstruction conversations are another central component of narrative therapy.

An example of applying ideas of deconstruction to therapeutic conversations

In order to explain how to apply ideas of deconstruction to therapeutic conversations, perhaps it is easiest to offer an example. In this case, let's consider two people who have come to consult a counsellor to talk about 'sexual difficulties' in their relationship. In this situation, both partners will come to therapy with particular beliefs and ideas about sexuality and relationships, influenced by the ideas of the culture in which they live. The couple may, for example, have particular ideas about how sex should be initiated or about what constitutes 'good' and 'bad' sexual experiences in relationships. The therapist can engage in explorations to identify some of the ideas and beliefs about sexuality that may be supporting the problem. There are many questions the therapist could ask to open a discussion of these:

- *What are some of your beliefs about people's roles in sexual/intimate relationships?*

- *What ideas do you have about what makes 'good' and 'bad' sexual experiences?*

- *How did these ideas develop?*

- *Are you comfortable with these ideas?*

- *Which ideas are helpful in your relationship? Which ones get in the way? How do they work against your relationship?*

Asking questions such as these is one way to open a deconstructing conversation. The therapist listens for any assumptions about life or relationships that may be in the interests of the problem and seeks to inquire about them. For example, either or both partners may be being influenced by particular assumptions as to what constitutes a 'healthy' relationship. These might be based on individualistic or gendered assumptions. The therapist may ask questions about the history of these beliefs and their effects on the life and relationships of the person consulting them.

When Jill and Jenny consulted a therapist about difficulties in their lesbian relationship, they identified the effects of homophobia and heterosexual dominance as contributing factors in their troubles. In deconstructive conversations, the therapist then explored with Jill and Jenny how heterosexist culture was negatively influencing their love and attraction for each other. These conversations uncovered how heterosexist notions about what constitutes a 'healthy relationship' were causing strain between Jill and Jenny. Incidents of homophobic violence and prejudice were also identified. By naming and unpacking some of these dominant cultural practices, Jenny and Jill were then able to explore how their relationship had been affected, and the history of these effects, and to consider the ways in which individually and together they had and could continue to create their own expressions of love.

Deconstructing Lucy's relationship with 'concentration'

Lucy consulted me about her difficulty with 'concentrating' on writing an important thesis. The problem was affecting many parts of Lucy's life. It had her thinking she was 'unproductive'. It tried to convince her that she would not be employable in the future, because if people saw her wandering around an office, not getting things done, they would think she was 'slack' or not worthy of a salary. The 'stress' was consuming her thoughts a lot of the time and affecting her physically – her stomach churned and she often felt sick and uncomfortable.

The voice of the problem was very critical and malicious, using sarcasm to try to convince her that she would never finish the thesis. It tried to tell her many things such as: 'You've approached it all the wrong way'; 'The method you've taken is all wrong'; 'You should be doing more with your day'; 'If you hadn't wasted so much time it would be done by now'; 'It has to be perfect, and just what the lecturer wants'.

She told me that the problem criticised her for making a cup of coffee or ringing a friend, as it told her that she was 'avoiding things' and that 'she would never get it finished'.

I asked Lucy about the problem's ideas on what constituted 'being productive'. In the course of the conversation we discovered that the problem had strict criteria. It thought that she should sit still in a chair for a fixed time period every day. During that time it thought she should only be thinking about the topic, and that she had to be either reading, typing, taking notes, or editing.

I opened a conversation that centred around where the problem got these ideas from about what is 'productive study'. This led to an exploration of the history of these ideas in Lucy's life. Lucy told me that these ideas about 'productive study' had been promoted throughout her school life and university career. Her earliest memory was during Grade 7 at school, when she was 11 years old. Since that time, Lucy told me that the ideas were supported by pamphlets and articles she had been given to read, talks she had attended on 'study skills' and conversations with her friends about studying.

I asked her about the effect of these ideas on her life – how she found them. Had she found them helpful or unhelpful? Lucy was certain that the ideas had distracted her and burdened her as she was always comparing her approach to their criteria and her ways never seemed good enough. Lucy thought the ideas had a negative effect on her view of herself as a student. She often felt worthless and incompetent, agitated and worried and as though she never 'measured up' to their expectations.

I discovered that Lucy had experienced some times away from the influence of these ideas. At these times she knew 'it will all work out. It's a bit of a challenge but it's fun and interesting, there will be an end,' and she experienced a confidence that 'I will find what I'm looking for'. Lucy said that when she broke from the problem's ideas about study, she knew that it was 'not the how' that was important. This led to a detailed discussion that concentrated

around specifying what 'not the how' meant to Lucy ('Not the how' became the alternative story which our subsequent conversations built upon.) We talked together about our knowledge of how artists 'work'. Lucy and I both shared what we knew of this – that many times an artist will just sit and think, drink a lot of coffee, make phone calls to friends, study colour combinations and experiment with mixing paints on their palettes. Many days could pass without the artist touching the canvas with paint. To an artist, it was 'not the how' that mattered, and artists often produced wonderful work as a result. We discussed other knowledges and experiences that also stood with the alternative story to open new possibilities for action for Lucy.

This conversation challenged the taken-for-granted truths and beliefs about study and assisted Lucy to break from the problem's ideas. It changed many things for Lucy – she was able to complete her writing and engaged in the project with more freedom and enjoyment. As I asked her about the problem's ideas on being productive and unproductive, I noticed Lucy seemed less burdened and she began to laugh at some of its ideas. This shift in the conversation assisted Lucy in breaking away from the dominant ideas towards an alternative story centred around her abilities, knowledge and skills as a student.

In this way, deconstruction can lead to the challenging of 'taken-for-granted' ideas and open alternative stories that assist people to challenge and break from the problem's views and to be more connected with their own preferred ideas, thoughts and ways of living.

Separating further from problems

When we examine the beliefs and ideas that may be supporting the life of a problem, we are assisting people to further separate from the problem. As we separate from these dominant ideas, we open new possibilities for challenging them and entering a new and preferred story or description. When this is done, people are assisted to break from the structures that sustain and support the problem. Often these conversations involve exploring considerations of gender, class, race and/or sexuality. These conversations shift the focus from the internalised processes of an individual to an externalised

focus on ideas and beliefs, the histories of these ideas and beliefs, their effects and different possibilities. As a result of these conversations people often feel freer from the influence of the ideas supporting the problem and this in itself alters their relationship to the problem and the problem story.

Deconstruction conversations help people to 'unpack' the dominant stories and view them from a different perspective. How these stories have been constructed becomes more visible. The dominant story becomes situated culturally and historically. These conversations often enable people to break further from a sense of guilt or blame as they come to see that the problem no longer speaks of their identity.

When the dominant ideas and beliefs that support the problem are exposed and discussed, times when the person has stood against or challenged them may also become visible. If this is significant to the person, it is a unique outcome that will open possibilities for the discovery of an alternative story. Once Lucy and I had explored the ideas of 'productive study' that had influenced her, the history of these ideas and their effects, Lucy felt more separate from them. Once separated, she began to laugh at them and what emerged were stories of times when the problem had had less influence upon her, times when her voice prevailed. Lucy thought these were significant and preferred, and they were thus unique outcomes to be further explored and developed (see chapter 7 on unique outcomes).

In deconstruction conversations it is important to note that therapists are not trying to impose their ideas or thoughts on the person, to 'change a person's thinking'. Nor are they imposing an outside point of view into the conversation. They are asking questions that they do not know the answers to, and they are remaining curious. They are inquiring as to the ideas and context that may be supporting the existence of the problem; they are tracing the history of these ideas, how they came into the person's life; they are asking questions that evaluate the effects of these beliefs, whether they are helpful or not. If these effects are judged not to be helpful, therapists are listening for unique outcomes – times when the person has acted in ways that indicate a breaking away from these dominant ideas. When these unique outcomes are identified, it is possible to explore them further as they are openings to alternative stories. This is considered in more detail in the following chapter.

Chapter 7

Discovering unique outcomes:
Listening for times when the problem has had less or no influence

As narrative therapists listen to the stories brought to therapy, they will hear of events that fit with the problem story and events that seem to contradict or stand outside of that dominant problem story. They will hear events that seem to fit with the influence of the problem, and events that stand against the problem's influence.

Josh and Tienne consulted a therapist interested in reclaiming their relationship from 'distance' and 'jealousy'. At their initial meeting they told the therapist about many events that fitted with this dominant description of their relationship. For instance, Tienne said: 'He just doesn't talk to me anymore, but he spends all his time either watching sport on TV and the only time we get to talk is when I go and turn it off. The other day he didn't come home from work until late and he just doesn't want to be with me.' Josh said: 'She won't tell me anything and when I ask her what is wrong she just shuts off and leaves the room. I can't seem to get through to her any more. She will only talk to her other friends. We used to share everything together.'

The therapist inquired about the times when they felt more connected to each other – before distance and jealousy interfered in their relationship. Tienne told the therapist about their enjoyment of bush walking and watching movies

together and Josh told the therapist about a sailing holiday that they had enjoyed some months previously. Tienne said: 'Well, we still go sailing together and that's not too bad. He sometimes will tell me things then and I'm always really surprised.' Josh agreed and offered 'Yes, we are always better if we have been sailing but that doesn't happen very often'. The therapist asked them what they would call this time they shared together, when they were sailing. Josh called it 'a closeness' and Tienne 'communication'.

When Josh and Tienne went sailing they experienced something different – a time away from the distance and jealousy. Both Josh and Tienne described this time as significant to them. Events like Josh and Tienne going sailing together, that are different or outside of the problem's influence, are known as unique outcomes.

A unique outcome can be anything that the problem would not like; anything that does not 'fit' with the dominant story. They are instances/events that would be difficult to achieve in the light of the problem. Josh and Tienne both thought that it was surprising to achieve communication and closeness whilst sailing and that this was difficult to achieve in the light of the dominant story (of a distant and jealous relationship). Narrative therapists would consider this a unique outcome and would be very interested to discover more about it. Sometimes unique outcomes are known as 'sparkling events' as they are like events that shine or stand out in contrast to the dominant story.

A unique outcome may be a plan, action, feeling, statement, quality, desire, dream, thought, belief, ability, or commitment. Unique outcomes can be in the past, the present and/or the future. Table 2 gives some examples of unique outcomes.

To begin with, I would suggest that therapists choose to focus their inquiry around a unique outcome that is very fresh in the recollections of the person(s), one that is very familiar to them. Generally, people find questions about these unique outcomes easier to answer, as they seem most relevant to their day-to-day experience of life, and this sort of inquiry is most likely to result in the rich description of an alternative story.

Table 2: Unique Outcomes

A plan: Mel planning to go out for a cup of coffee when Anorexia tries to tell her she will get fat and shouldn't go. (past)

An action: Ari ringing a friend when the voice of depression has tried to isolate him from his friends. (past)

A feeling: Marcy feeling pleased with her exam results when Self-Perfectionism tried to tell her they weren't good enough. (present)

A statement: Paula giving her opinions in a meeting when Self-Doubt tried to silence her. (past)

A quality: Erin maintaining her care for others in the face of abusive practices in her work environment. (present)

A desire/dream: Dave hoping to share a holiday with his family when his life is free of the influence of alcohol and drugs. (future)

A thought: Xiang thinking 'It's not my fault' when mother blaming tried to talk her into feeling responsible for her daughter being subject to abuse. (present and past)

A belief: Luz saying ' I believe I will get better from this' when Depression tries to tell him that this is impossible. (present)

An ability: Chris and Leanne laughing together about something their daughter had said to them. 'Expectations' had on many occasions got between them and made it difficult for them to experience joy with parenting. (present)

A commitment: Roberto and Laurie being committed to non-violent forms of parenting when their own experience had been one of abuse. (past and present)

Discovering unique outcomes

Unique outcomes may be discovered during therapeutic conversations as well as during the times between, before and after these conversations. Many people I have spoken to consider the act of making an appointment and coming to speak with a therapist about a problem as a significant unique outcome. Speaking about a problem with another person usually represents a stand against a problem's influence. I asked Asha, 'Did anxiety try to stop you from coming today?' Asha told me of many times when anxiety had stopped her from phoning to make an appointment and that it was a 'big thing' to arrive at my office and not to 'back out at the last minute, like I usually do'.

During a conversation, the therapist may notice events that stand outside the problem story. Nic and his family consulted me about the effects of an 'Attention Deficit Disorder' diagnosis. During our meeting Nic sat quite still and attentive in a chair for 30 minutes out of the 60 minute session. This ability caught my attention as being different from what ADD would want. When I asked about this, Nic and his sister told me that 'Yes, that is good for Nic but he can sit still when he is in Art class or when 'Rug Rats' is on television'. ('Rug Rats' is a popular children's cartoon program.)

Once the history and effects of the problem have been traced, the therapist is listening for any times when the problem had less, little or no influence over the person. They are on the look-out for times that are exceptions or different from the dominant problem-saturated story. As the therapist inquires about a particular unique outcome, other times free from the problem's influence become more apparent/visible/accessible/available. Noticing Nic's ability to sit still in the session led me to discover some other times when ADD did not interrupt his life. As these unique outcomes are explored further, they were be linked and joined together, to form a new and alternative story, separate from the ADD story.

Unique outcomes (events that stand outside of the dominant story or problem) can often go unnoticed, unless the therapist listens and watches out for them. People tend to place less significance on these events and will often mention them very quickly or in passing. They can pass through a conversation without being commented upon unless they are noticed by the therapist and inquired about. Unique outcomes might be mentioned incidentally. It is up to

the therapist to pay particular attention to them.

The therapist is interested in an inquiry of these events as they can serve as openings to richer descriptions of the lives and relationships of the people seeking counselling. Unique outcomes can be doorways to alternative stories. If we consider the diagram below (figure 2), unique outcomes can be thought of as the Xs outside those events connected with the dominant story. Whilst they are less visible in the light of the dominant story, they are nonetheless there, ready to be discovered.

Figure 2

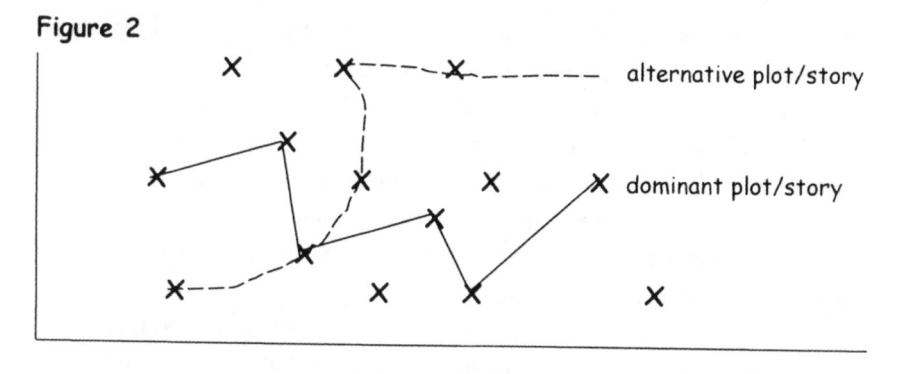

Therapists influenced by narrative ways of working assume that these events or unique outcomes do not exist in isolation. They assume that problems are never 100% successful and that, therefore, there will be other events across time that can be traced and linked with the unique outcome that has been discovered. Narrative therapists do not see these times, these unique outcomes, as a fluke, nor do they put them down to chance. They consider these sparkling events to be openings to a new and different conversation – openings to escape the thin conclusions and to move towards richer descriptions.

There are many other ways to discover unique outcomes. When a therapist meets with a family and traces the history of the problem and the effects of the problem in the family's life, they hear about many events that fit with the dominant story. Throughout these explorations, however, they remain curious about any events that do not fit with the dominant story.

When inquiring about the effects of Self-Hate on her relationships with friends, Suzanne reported: 'Oh no, I still go out and meet with my friends … Self-hate doesn't stop me from doing that, I wouldn't let it.' This ability seemed to be an exception or something different from the dominant story of Self-Hate.

It is important to note, however, that such events are not unique outcomes until the therapist consults the person as to their significance. This is most important. It is up to the person who is seeking counselling to determine whether something is or is not a unique outcome. The therapist must ask the person about the event to check whether or not they consider it to be special and unique. If they do consider it as different and significant, and a contradiction to the dominant story, then and only then can it be considered a unique outcome. A trap that therapists can fall into is to identify these times away from the dominant story, to evaluate them as significant and as a result get in a position of trying to convince the person that the event is significant. This often leads the therapist into a position of 'pointing out positives' and is not the approach that narrative therapists are interested in. An event that stands outside of the dominant story is only a unique outcome if the person consulting the therapist judges it to be so. Careful enquiry and consultation assists the therapist to always leave evaluating the significance of certain events as unique outcomes to the person whose life is being discussed.

The therapist can ask direct questions to discover the significance of an event that they suspect may be a unique outcome: 'What does it mean to you that Self-Hate hasn't got in the way of your friendships? Does that stand out to you?' Sometimes the therapist may notice events that seem to stand outside the effects of the dominant problem story and hesitantly inquire about them: 'I was just thinking that when you meet your friends, it seems like you are going against the Self-Hates rules in some way? What do you think? Does that seem important or not?' Similarly the therapist might ask 'How did that seem to you? Did it surprise you or not surprise you that you did this?' Sometimes the significance of the event for the person is easier to determine by noticing changes in emotion or body language. The way in which the person is speaking may give the therapist a clue. The person's tone of voice might shift towards being more excited or relieved, their body posture may become more relaxed or at ease, their facial expressions happy or brighter perhaps. These shifts in emotion during the session give the therapist some clues as to the significance the person places on the event.

The significance of certain events can also be determined by something the person may say, such as: 'I couldn't believe I went through with booking the ticket for the holiday. I've tried so many times to do that but just didn't have the

guts, but I just did it and didn't even have to think about it.' People's expressions often tell the therapist how they have judged the event: however, it is still sometimes necessary for the therapist to clarify the event's importance. Listening for these expressions is therefore important.

In some circumstances where the person consulting the therapist may be very captured by the problem story, the unique outcome may seem very small. There is no need for a unique outcome to be large or spectacular in any way. What will become significant, if the person determines that it is indeed a unique outcome, are the ways in which the unique outcome is understood and described and the ways it is linked to other events and meanings.

The therapist may need to be very curious about a particular event and tease out what made its occurrence possible. To begin with, the person whose life is being discussed may not see the event as particularly significant. The therapist may ask some questions about the event before they ask the person to evaluate its significance. If the therapist asks the person to evaluate the possible unique outcome too early, without an exploration of the context of the event, or the obstacles that could have prevented the particular action taking place, it may reduce the meaningfulness of the event. The therapist therefore tries to create a context that enables the person to more easily appreciate the significance of a particular event. However, and this is very important, the therapist should never presume to know how any person has experienced a particular event. It is ultimately up to the person themselves to make a judgement as to the significance or lack of significance of any particular event. It is up to the person(s) consulting the therapist to determine whether or not a certain event, thought, act, belief, ability or commitment contradicts the dominant story to such an extent that it is considered significant and therefore a unique outcome.

Back-up questions

In situations in which the therapist for some reason is unable to find an entry point to explore possible unique outcomes, there are some 'back-up' questions that a therapist may consider using.

• *How have you managed to stop the problem from getting worse?*

• *Are there times when the problem is not as bad as usual? Are there times*

when it is less dominating and bossy?

- *Can you think of a time when the problem could have stopped you or got in the way, but didn't? What happened?*

- *Is there a story you could tell me about a time when you resisted the problem and did what you wanted to do instead?*

Relative influence questions (see chapter 4) can also be used as a back-up to discover unique outcomes. If a person has judged the problem to have 80% of their life, the therapist may consider asking about the 20% that they have managed to maintain.

To discover unique outcomes, I would encourage therapists to rely more on their skills in listening and attending than on these back-up questions. When a unique outcome is identified in the course of the conversation, it is often experienced by the person as far more helpful than if they were asked a back-up question.

Summary

In summary, when meeting with people, narrative therapists are interested in bringing forth a new or different story about people's lives and relationships. The beginnings of these stories are times or events that do not fit with, or are contrary to, the dominant story. It is assumed that a problem will never be 100% successful in claiming a person's life. There will always be exceptions or times of difference. These times of difference are known as unique outcomes. Anything that defies the problem or that contravenes the problem can be seen as a unique outcome or sparkling event – if so identified by the person concerned. These are times when the problem has less, little or no influence over the person's life. These may be times, beliefs, events, thoughts, feelings, actions or ideas that stand outside of the influence of the problem. These are the openings for new and different stories to be discovered.

Further reading

White, M. 1995: 'The narrative perspective in therapy.' In White, M., *Re-authoring Lives: Interviews and essays,* chapter 1. Adelaide: Dulwich Centre Publications.

Chapter 8

Tracing the history and meaning of the unique outcome and naming an alternative story

As therapists discover unique outcomes they are interested in exploring them further, tracing their history and understanding what they mean to the person concerned. Unique outcomes are the doorways or openings to new and different stories.

The therapist attempts to trace the history of the unique outcomes, firmly ground them, make them more visible, and link them in some way with an emerging new story. As more and more unique outcomes are traced, grounded, linked and given meaning, a new plot emerges and an alternative story becomes more richly described. By paying attention to the unique outcomes, the therapist facilitates the placing of these events more in the foreground of people's consciousness/awareness. Attributing meaning to them and linking them to other events in the past contributes powerfully to the co-authoring of a new story. This alternative story is usually 'anti-problem' and brings forth people's skills, abilities, competencies and commitments. Identifying some of these competencies may have been difficult when they were overshadowed by the dominant problem story, and the act of bringing them forward assists people to reconnect with their preferences, hopes, dreams and ideas. Bringing the alternative story forth and accessing people's skills and abilities will, it is assumed, in turn affect future actions. Throughout this process the therapist

consults the person about the emerging story, how it suits their life and how it fits with their preferences for living.

Exploring the particularities of the unique outcome

When therapists first discover an event, thought, action, belief, idea, dream or hope that does not fit with the dominant story, they are interested in discovering as much information and detail as they can about it. Their questions often will begin with Who? What? Where? When? so that the particularities of the unique outcome can be explored in detail.

The therapist wants to understand as much as possible about the event – each small detail. These questions explore what is known as the landscape of action.[4]

> *The landscape of action is constituted by experiences of events that are liked together in sequences through time and according to specific plots. This provides us with the rudimentary structure of stories. If we drop one of those dimensions out – experiences of events, sequences, time, or plot – then we wouldn't have a story. These events together, make up the landscape of action.* (White 1995, p.31)

Landscape of action questions

Here are some examples of landscape of action questions which therapists may ask as they are exploring a unique outcome:

- *Where were you when this happened?*
- *Were you on your own or with someone else?*
- *When did it happen?*
- *How long did it last?*
- *What happened just before and after?*

---

[4] This term was first developed by Jerome Bruner (1986). It was introduced to the therapy field by Michael White (1991).

- *How did you prepare yourself?*
- *What did your friend say when you told him?*
- *Was it a decision you made on your own or with someone?*
- *Have you done this before or was this the first time?*
- *What were the steps leading up to doing this?*

In this way, landscape of action questions involve inquiries not only into the details of the particular unique outcome but also into any other actions and events that may be linked to the unique outcome. Questions might be asked about any events/actions that led up to the unique outcome, events/actions that occurred just after it, or events/actions from the distant past that could be linked in some way to the unique outcome that is being discussed.

Exploring the meaning of the unique outcome

The person consulting the therapist is then invited to reflect on the meanings of the events or unique outcomes that they have described. This interpretation or giving of meaning is likely to cement the unique outcome into a foundation of other events across time. An exploration is undertaken into what the development (unique outcome) means in terms of the person's desires, intentions, preferences, beliefs, hopes, personal qualities, values, strengths, commitments, plans, characteristics, abilities, and purposes. These questions are known as landscape of identity questions (again this term was originally used by Jerome Bruner, see above).

As they talk about certain events they will indicate what they think those events reflect about the character, motives, desires and so on, of various persons in their social networks. They will also reflect upon what these events say about the qualities of particular relationships. So, the landscape of identity or meaning has to do with the interpretations that are made through reflection on those events that are unfolding through landscapes of action. (White 1995, p.31)

Landscape of identity⁵ questions

Here are some examples of landscape of identity questions.

Desires, wishes, preferences:

- *When you agreed to go out with your friends for dinner, what do you think that says about what you want for your life?*

- *Staying in contact with your lecturer in your course – what does that say about what is important for your life?*

- *What do you think that says about the hopes you have for your relationship with your daughter?*

Personal values:

- *What personal values is this course of action based upon?*

- *When you rang your grandmother after the argument, what did that mean for/about what you value in your relationship? What personal values does this show?*

Relationship qualities:

- *When that happened, how would you describe your relationship with John at that time?*

Personal skills and abilities:

- *What went into doing this at this point in your life?*

- *What did it take in order to do this?*

Intentions, motives, plans, purposes:

- *When you took this step what were you intending for your life?*

- *What does it say about what you were planning?*

---

⁵ Landscape of identity questions are sometimes referred to as landscape of consciousness questions.

- *What does it say about you as a person that you would do this?*

Beliefs and values:

- *Managing to stay working in a pathologising setting, using respectful ideas – what does that say about what you think is important?*

- *Can you help me understand more about what that says you believe in or value?*

Personal qualities:

- *What does it say about you as a person that you would do this?*

- *What did it take for you to do that?*

- *What do you think that says about your abilities/skills/knowledges?*

There is no particular order in which to ask these sorts of questions. The therapist may ask about the details of the events and then switch to inquire about what these events mean in terms of the person's interests or beliefs. The therapist might ask first about the details and then the meanings. These questions are woven back and forth, in and out, assisting to creating a new and different story.

> *In re-authoring work we invite persons to traffic in both of these landscapes* [action and identity] *– by reflecting on what alternative events in the landscape of action might mean, and by determining which events in the landscape of action most reflect the preferred accounts of characteristics, of motive, of belief and so on – so that alternative landscapes of action and of identity are brought forth.* (White 1995, p.31)

Creating a new story

Melanie (8 years) consulted me about her relationships with her peers. 'Fights and arguments' were getting in the way of her friendship with Rebecca and were creating a space between them that did not suit Melanie. This space sometimes meant that Melanie and Rebecca would not speak to each other, even when their families spent time together on weekends. Melanie was interested in getting her friendship back from 'fights and arguments'. In one of our conversations, Melanie told me of an event that had recently occurred. She said that she felt so strongly that she had 'had enough' that she just went straight up to Rebecca and said 'This is ridiculous, we have to start talking because it is ruining everything'. Melanie considered this to be a particularly sparkling moment. She was rather shocked that she had taken this action considering that the two girls had not spoken for several weeks due to the influence of 'fights and arguments'. This unique outcome prompted me to ask Melanie many landscape of action and landscape of identity questions in order to place this development in an alternative story about their relationship. This alternative story was judged to be preferred by Melanie and Rebecca. To give you an idea of how this type of conversation might sound I will share part of a conversation and some of the questions I asked Melanie.

Each question in the following transcript has been given a number that relates to the diagram below. This diagram shows how the landscape of identity and landscape of action questions are woven back and forth in my conversation with Melanie, as I follow the details that she offers in relation to significance of the unique outcome.

Conversation between Alice & Melanie

Landscape of Action Questions (about the details of the unique outcomes)

1 — 2 — 3 — 4 — 5   7 — 8   12 (both)   15 (both)   18

                    6   9 — 10 — 11   12 — 13 — 14   15 — 16 — 17

Landscape of Identity Questions (that derive the meaning of the event)

Question 1

Alice: So you actually went up to Rebecca and said that, is that right?

Melanie: Yes.

Question 2

Alice: Can you tell me a bit more about it, like where were you both? At school or at Rebecca's house, at your house? Where did this happen?

Melanie: It happened on the way to the library. We were just walking along so I just thought I'd say it.

Question 3

Alice: And what led up to this? How did you prepare yourself to do this?

Melanie: Well, I went to Rebecca's on the weekend and my little brother was really sad because he wanted to play with Rebecca's brother and he couldn't because Rebecca and I don't talk. I have been thinking since then that it just has to stop because it is messing up everyone's life, not just Rebecca's and my life.

Question 4

Alice: How many days were you thinking about it before you said this?

Melanie: Oh ... about four or five days.

Question 5

Alice: And how much thinking did you do about it? A lot or just a little bit or what would you say?

Melanie: Oh, a lot because it was hard to go to sleep because I was thinking about it so much and I couldn't do my school work as well as I usually can.

Question 6

Alice: So would you say that you were the sort of person who prefers to sort things out? Is that something that you stand for as a person?

Melanie: Yes. I think it's important to try to work things out with people.

Question 7

Alice: And so what happened then?

Melanie: Well, Rebecca said that she agreed that it had been going on too long and she said she wanted to be friends too.

Question 8
Alice: What else did she say, can I ask you?
Melanie: She told me she was glad that I talked to her because she didn't have the 'guts' to do it.

Question 9
Alice: So Rebecca thought it took a lot of courage or bravery to do this? Would you agree or do you think it took something else?
Melanie: Oh yes! It was bravery because before I was really nervous and I had to just be brave to come out and say it.

Question 10
Alice: So when you were doing all this thinking and then spoke to Rebecca, what do you think that says about what you think is important between Rebecca and you?
Melanie: It's important to try to work things out with people. And I really want to be Rebecca's friend.

Question 11
Alice: So you are the type of person who values working things out, and values your friendship with Rebecca. Is that what you are saying?
Melanie: Yes ... because then everyone can have more fun.

Question 12
Alice: So when you were thinking since the weekend about Rebecca and you, can you tell me some more about that thinking? Was it to do with your values in working things out or your interest in everyone having fun or your desire to have Rebecca as your friend or something else?
Melanie: Yes, it was all of that and I was just thinking that Rebecca and I used to be such good friends and did so much together and I thought that if we could talk about it we might work something out and make it fair to everyone.

Question 13

Alice: Is fairness something you would say you stand for too?

Melanie: Yes, I think being fair is really important if you are going to be someone's friend.

Question 14

Alice: What other things do you think talking to Rebecca like you did says about what is important to you in your friendships?

Melanie: I think it's important to speak kindly to your friends.

Question 15

Alice: So how did you speak with Rebecca that day? Did you use your 'speaking kindly' skills to help you or something else?

Melanie: I used them but also I thought 'How would I want someone to talk to me?' And that's how I talked to Rebecca.

Question 16

Alice: So, talking like you would like to be talked to – what would you say that means about what you believe in or what you intend for your friendships?

Melanie: Well, I want my friends to always talk to me like that too.

Question 17

Alice: Is there a name for this way of talking to your friends that you are committed to?

Melanie: Well it's fairness and kind talking.

Question 18

Alice: This fair and kind talking, is it something new or have you had this commitment for a long time?

Melanie: A long time.

In this way an alternative story is named as 'fairness and kind talking'. Earlier, a plot of bravery could also have built upon, but as the problem involved fighting and conflict, it seemed more appropriate to focus on an alternative story of fairness and kindness. When I asked Melanie, she said that

she preferred this name.

Identifying the unique outcome, and using landscape of action and landscape of identity questions, leads to an exploration of Melanie's values, commitments, beliefs, desires, intentions and strengths. These are articulated and brought into the foreground of an emerging alternative story. As they are articulated, Melanie is assisted in reconnecting with them. As she reconnects with them and they are firmly planted and explored across time, they can be linked to other events that fit with this new story. These preferences are brought to the foreground, placing the dominant problematic story of their relationship more towards the background. The questions have brought forward a rich description of Melanie's abilities to act in relation to the problem's influence – her personal agency.

Through these questions I inquired about the near past – the preparations that led up to this unique outcome. I could also explore this development in the more distant past to discover some more about the history of some of these commitments and strengths. Questions can bring forth other events in the alternative story that are linked to this unique outcome: 'Is this commitment to fairness something new for you or is this something that you have stood for for a long time? How long? Could you tell me something about what you know about this bravery? When did you first notice this strength? Have you used it at other times or is this the first time? These questions help to ground the unique outcome across time, in accordance with the new plot.

I can also ask her about the implications of these commitments, beliefs, strengths and desires, in the future: 'How will your commitment to fairness, working things out together and kind talking effect your friendships in the future? What effect would you say these beliefs and intentions and personal qualities might have on your friendship with Rebecca from now on?' Melanie thought that it would assist them to gain back their relationship even further from fights and arguments and 'make them even closer best friends'.

These commitments, strengths, beliefs and desires are now resources that are more accessible to Melanie in the present and the future. If the dominant story (fights and arguments) attempts a comeback, these resources will assist Melanie to stay connected with her preferences for her relationship with Rebecca. Discussing these resources will affect Melanie's future actions and shape her life from here.

Other avenues for the rich description of skills and abilities

Sometimes questions that draw out rich descriptions of personal skills, commitments, beliefs and values can be asked 'through the eyes of another person'. The other person chosen should be someone dear to, or respected by, the person. This person can be identified in a number of ways. The therapist's knowledge of the person may assist. They may know, for example, that the person consulting them holds the opinions of their teacher, grandparent, parent, friend, cartoon character, movie character, or relative in high esteem. The therapist's knowledge about the person would assist them to ask a question like, 'If your grandmother had witnessed you speaking to Rebecca that way, what do you think she would say about the type of person you are, the sorts of qualities you have as a person?'

Another way to discover who might be able to offer a significant reflection is by asking questions such as: 'Who would be least surprised that you did this or thought this? What might they say about this? What would they know about you that would not make them surprised? What personal skills could they tell me about that would have them not surprised? What would they say this says about what you want for your life?'

Later chapters will explore more fully these sorts of questions (which Michael White refers to as re-membering questions).

Naming an alternative story

Earlier chapters have described the process of naming the problem, exploring its effects, evaluating these effects and inviting a justification of this evaluation. We have now also considered ways of initially noticing and exploring the significance of unique outcomes and how this contributes to the creation of an alternative, non-problematic story or narrative. Just as there may be many different problems to externalise, there may also be a variety of alternative stories. In Melanie's situation, as described above, two options included 'bravery' and 'fairness and kind talking'.

It is important that the person consulting the therapist does this naming.

Again, as with the naming of the dominant problem story, the therapist may offer tentative suggestions, using the words of the person consulting them, but the crucial factor is that the name for the alternative story is derived from the person's own words and experience.

Various questions can assist the process of coming up with a name for the alternative story, including:

- *What would you call this project that involves standing up to the effects of harassment?*

- *When you talk about 'making your life your own', would this be a good name for us to use for what you want more of?*

- *Is 'holding onto hope' a fair way of describing this other way of doing things, that is resisting depression's grip on your life?*

Using the statement of position map with alternative stories

Just as in relation to naming the problem, it is possible to ask people to explore the effects of the alternative story or counter-plot, to evaluate these effects, and to ask people to justify this evaluation (see chapter 5). This further use of the statement of position map allows a consolidation of the counter-plot and an articulation of its effects (both actual effects in the present and those that may become possible in the future). It also enables the therapist to check that the counter-plot being articulated is a preferred direction for the person and why it is important to them. This opens possibilities to thicken the alternative story.

Dorothy's strength and survival in the face of 'worthlessness'

Dorothy first came to therapy with a story about herself as being a victim of rape, a damaged person, and someone who was incapable of sustaining relationships with men. As she discussed her concerns with the therapist, the problem was externalised as 'worthlessness'. Through these externalising conversations, certain sparkling events and thoughts in Dorothy's life came to

the attention of the therapist who was interested in exploring them further. Dorothy said she was also surprised about these events and was interested in talking more about three new developments that had occurred recently.

Firstly, she had accepted a dinner invitation a few days previously, from a man, and had not felt scared about going. Secondly, she had begun to think differently about the rape ('I used to think that I was to blame but now I think that it was him who had the problem'). And thirdly, she had been experiencing less of the frightening 'flash-backs' that had been a part of her life since the rape. She also told the therapist that the rape had not negatively affected her work or certain aspects of her social life and that she had been surprised at how, over the past few months, she had been able to speak about the rape with a friend of hers. These events stood outside of the 'worthless' person story that had been a dominant description for Dorothy for some years. Dorothy was interested in these new developments continuing as they were contributing to her experiencing her life more positively.

The therapist asked Dorothy about her understanding of the meaning of these thoughts and events. Dorothy said she thought they meant that she was a 'strong person and a survivor, who wanted to get on with her life'. As Dorothy and the therapist further explored this emerging new story of strength and survival, other events and thoughts that fitted with the new story were discovered. 'Strength and survival' became the title or name for Dorothy's alternative story. It was a story that stood in stark contrast to the problem-saturated description she had first arrived with.

When Dorothy was asked to explore the effects of this alternative story, she said that 'strength and survival' made her feel as if her life was her life, and that they made her feel safe and more secure in the world. When asked to evaluate these effects, Dorothy said that they were good effects and that she wanted more of those feelings in her life. When asked why this was so, Dorothy said that it was such a long time since she felt safe in the world and that she longed to feel secure and hoped to become independent again so that her family would no longer need to support her. She also wished that one day she would feel confident in having children of her own.

In this way the alternative story was named 'strength and survival' and the statement of position map was used to more richly describe it by linking it to the landscape of identity to Dorothy's hopes and dreams.

Why name the alternative story?

Finding a name for the alternative story brings many advantages. The process itself can assist people to further separate from the effects of the dominant story and allow space to consider their own ideas and commitments. Personal preferences and choices become more visible, and this can make it easier for people to create more of what they would like. Naming both the alternative story and the dominant story provides a framework with which all future events or actions can be mapped. These names or plot lines are useful as constant points of reference in future conversations. Once they are named, the therapist can consult the person about whether any action or event fits more with the dominant story (e.g. 'worthlessness) or the alternative one (e.g. 'strength and survival'). A question may sound something like this: 'Melanie, when you said that to Rebecca, would you say it fitted more with "fights and arguments" or with "fairness and kind talking"?' When people are asked to answer such questions, they are invited into choice and selection based upon their personal preferences – a process that makes them agents for their own lives, authoring their own stories.

Once an alternative story has been named, the therapist is interested in how this story can become more richly described. There are many different ways that this can occur and the possibilities will be explored in the next few chapters.

Further reading

White, M. 1991: 'Deconstruction and therapy.' *Dulwich Centre Newsletter*, No.3. Reprinted in Epston, D. & White, M. (1992), *Experience, Contradiction, Narrative & Imagination*. Adelaide: Dulwich Centre Publications.

White, M. 1995: 'The narrative perspective in therapy.' In White, M., *Re-authoring Lives: Interviews & essays*. Adelaide: Dulwich Centre Publications.

Part Two

Thickening
the
alternative story

Introduction

As a new and preferred story begins to emerge, the therapist is interested in finding ways to assist the person consulting them to 'hold onto' or stay connected to it. Staying connected with the emerging alternative story can be a challenge for many people. For example, as Dorothy's new story of 'strength and survival' begins to emerge (as described in the previous chapter), the therapist would be mindful that it was likely to be difficult for Dorothy to hold onto this new description of herself without some support. This is understandable as the dominant story of 'worthlessness' had been shaping and influencing her life for many years. In this situation, the therapist would be interested in thinking of ways to assist Dorothy to keep this emerging story close to her in her daily life. Therapists engaged with narrative ways of working would assume that when Dorothy is more connected to this new story it will assist her in the present as well as shape her future actions. As Dorothy indicated that this new story is a positive direction for her, consistent with her preferences, hopes and values for living, the therapist would wish to find ways of thickening this story, of making it more richly described and thus more available to Dorothy. It would be the therapist's role to provide some structured ways for Dorothy to stay connected to the story of herself as strong, and as a survivor.

One way of thickening the alternative story involves finding witnesses who will act as an audience to performances of the new story. Therapists are therefore interested in trying to engage audiences to the emerging alternative story. If the therapist can find ways in which the people in this audience can not only act as witnesses, but can link their lives in some way to the new story of the person consulting the therapist, this can significantly add life and richness to this new story.

There are many possibilities for inviting an audience to engage with the alternative story. The audience may consist of people, present or absent from the session, real or imaginary, from the person's past or present.

Some of the ways in which other people are engaged in this part of the work include:

- through re-membering conversations (chapter 9)

- as members of leagues, networks, committees, groups, or teams and co-research (chapter 13)

- as participants within rituals and celebrations (chapter 12)

- in definitional ceremonies as outsider-witness group members or as members of reflecting teams (chapter 14)

There are also other options for thickening the alternative story that do not necessarily involve other people directly. These include:

- therapeutic documentation – including declarations, documents, certificates, handbooks, notes from the session, videotapes, symbols, lists and pictures (chapter 10)

- therapeutic letters (chapter 11)

All of these options can play their part in creating a richer description of the alternative story and this in turn can assist the person consulting the therapist to stay connected with the new preferred story. The therapist and Dorothy might choose to use one, two, or perhaps more of these options over the course of their meetings. The choice will depend upon a number of things: Dorothy's interest, her skills (for example reading and writing abilities), her preferences (some people prefer visual media, other auditory, others written), the availability of other people, the time available (for example to write a letter or phone a person), accessibility, (for example, outsider-witness groups are usually made up of two or more people), the therapist's interests/skills, the therapist's knowledge of the person and of their likes and dislikes, the therapist's understanding of the person's past experiences and what would fit for them, and/or the knowledge the therapist has gained from others in similar situations about what is helpful.

The possibilities are almost endless in this area of the work. The following chapters will explore the different options in some detail.

Chapter 9

Re-membering
conversations

To understand what is meant by re-membering conversations, it is first necessary to think about a person's life as a club with members. When we think about all those people whom we are associated with in the course of our daily lives, we could consider them as members of our 'club' of life. Some of these members we may have consciously invited into our lives, others we may have had little choice over including. Re-membering conversations involve people deliberately choosing who they would like to have more present as the members of their club of life, and whose memberships they would prefer to revise or revoke. The use of the term re-membering is therefore not just about recollecting or being reminded. The hyphen between re and membering is significant to its meaning and use in narrative therapy.[6]

When people are faced with a problem, they often experience isolation and disconnection from important relationships. The dominant problem story may be successful in minimising or making invisible certain partnerships or histories in the person's life. Re-membering conversations are intended to redress this and powerfully incorporate and elevate significant people's contribution in the lives of those consulting the therapist. Engaging in these

---

[6] The term re-membering was coined by Barbara Myerhoff (1982). It was introduced into the therapy world by Michael White (1997).

conversations provides a direct contrast to many current cultural practices that encourage individualisation and disconnection of people from one another.

When the therapist begins to discover an event or events that stand outside of the problem's influence (unique outcomes) they are curious to discover as much as possible about them. They trace the history of these events and attempt to locate them amongst other events outside of the problem's influence (landscape of action questions). As these events are linked in a history over time, people are invited to explore their meanings: what these events mean in terms of their personal qualities, commitments, preferences, desires, beliefs, skills, knowledge, etc. (landscape of identity questions). As these are linked into an alternative story, and as the alternative story is given a name and more thoroughly explored, the therapist wonders:

- *Who else would know about this?*

- *Who else would know what this person stands for? [outside of the problem's influence]*

- *Who would be least surprised to hear them say this?*

The therapist wonders this because they are trying to identify other people who may be knowledgeable about this different story of the person's identity. It is likely that these memberships are hidden from the awareness of the person and the therapist is interested in bringing them forward and making them more visible. Therapists assume that identifying these significant people will further add to the identity description and alternative story that is being generated.

Re-membering conversations can contribute significantly to richly describing the history of alternative stories. Significant figures in a person's life are often the holders of memories of events in which the person consulting the therapist displayed certain skills, traits and abilities. The significant person's knowledge of these events can be linked with other events in the alternative story that is being generated. Linking together events in the alternative story in this way contributes to rich description.

Significant memberships may include people alive or no longer living; they may be related or unrelated to the person, real or imaginary, from their past or present. These memberships may also include animals, toys, pets, places,

symbols or objects. All these possibilities can be explored widely.

The therapist may ask the people consulting them questions to discover these memberships:

- *Who would be least surprised to hear you say this?*

- *Who else would know that you stand for tolerance and peace?*

- *Is there someone you can think of who could tell a story about you in relation to your commitment to loving relationships?*

- *Can you think of someone who would know something about your preference for parenting in this way?*

- *If I wanted to discover some more about this skill of yours, who (other than you) would be able to tell me about it?*

One or more memberships may be identified. The therapist continues to be curious about what these people would say about the person and their history. The therapist would ask many questions to explore what these people would be likely to know and say. A question in these conversations could be: 'If your aunt [the significant member identified] was here today and I was able to ask her a little about you, what do you think she would tell me about these skills of yours? When would she have first noticed them?'

The therapist would continue to ask questions to invite speculation about what the significant member would be thinking, what would have led them to these ideas, when they first would have thought this, what they would say, why they would say this, etc. Questions that begin with Who, What, Where, When, How and Why can extract rich descriptions of these significant details. The therapist might also ask questions about what the person's relationship with the significant member would have meant for them. For example: 'What do you think it meant for your aunt for you to include her in your life in this way? What do you think it meant for her to spend those times with you?'

Through these sorts of conversations, an historical alternative account of the person's identity can be generated and the significant memberships of a person's life can begin to be privileged and explored. The therapist assumes that this is helpful in itself but sometimes it may be possible for the person to actually re-connect with these re-membered people in other ways.

The therapist may try to contact these people and interview them about

their knowledge of the person who is consulting the therapist (see Sonia's ritual of membership described in chapter 12). Letters, phone calls, emails or invitations to meet are often extended to the people identified so that the therapist can discover more about these aspects of the person's identity that relate to the alternative stories of their lives (see chapter 11). This will thicken these accounts and add to the story of identity that the therapist and the person at the centre of the therapy are co-authoring. These meetings with significant others are often extremely important in the course of the therapy. They engage people with a history to the alternative story that is linked to the lives of others in ways that powerfully contradict the problem-saturated account of their lives.

If significant people identified in these conversations are unable to be contacted, if they are no longer alive or are unable to communicate, sometimes someone who was or is close to the significant person can act as a stand-in. In these situations, the therapist can ask a series of questions to the person who is standing in, who then endeavours to give answers 'through the eyes' of the significant person.

In the following examples I detail just a few of the many possibilities for re-membering conversations.

Sophia

Sophia (aged six years) was reclaiming her sleep from the influence of bad dreams. She had been successful in having four nights of happy dreams when I met with her and her Baby Born doll. Sophia told me that she had managed to reclaim her sleep by doing some 'hard thinking'. After ensuring that abuse was not a part of the context of Sophia's life, I was interested in further exploring Sophia's skills in addressing the bad dreams. I asked her if 'hard thinking' was something she had always had, or something new. Sophia was not sure. I pursued my interest in her skill further with the assistance of re-membering questions. If I had not, this skill in the alternative story would have gone unnoticed and disappeared. The rich description of this skill might not have been articulated and explored and this would have closed the door on many of the unique discoveries that were subsequently made.

I asked Sophia if there was anyone who would not be surprised that she

was 'a hard thinker'. Sophia did not know. I then named some possibilities for her, from my knowledge of relationships in her life:

Alice: Would your mum or your dad or your teacher, grandma, cousin, friend, or maybe one of your toys know anything about this ability of yours to use hard thinking?

Sophia: (after a pause) I think Baby Born [a toy] and mummy would know a little bit.

Alice: If I were to ask them about it, what would they tell me?

Sophia: I don't know what mummy would say but Baby Born would know because she sees me do my homework.

Alice: What does she see you do?

Sophia: She sees me thinking hard when something is hard.

Alice: So you think hard when things are hard and are you the sort of person who gives up or keeps going? What would Baby Born say about that?

Sophia: She would say that I never give up when things are hard because I know my four times tables and that was hard and I didn't give up.

Alice: So what would Baby Born call that quality you have in not giving up when things get hard?

Sophia: A fighter

From this brief conversation further qualities of 'being a fighter' and 'sticking to things' were identified. This led to me asking many more questions about the history of these qualities and about other members of Sophia's life who would also know about them. In this way these qualities were richly and thickly described. Once more richly described, these abilities and accounts of Sophia's identity would be more available for Sophia in the future. I believed this would help her with the bad dreams and would ripple out to benefit other parts of her life as well.

Sophia was unsure of what her mother would know about her hard thinking. I guessed that she might know something that might be interesting to find out about, so I suggested inviting Sophia's mother, Marcia, to join us for a

meeting. At this meeting I interviewed Marcia in Sophia's presence about her knowledge of Sophia's hard thinking skills, her fighting spirit, and her ability to stick to things when they are hard. Many more stories of these abilities emerged, adding to a new story of Sophia's identity. This process enabled Sophia to break from the bad dreams. It also made it possible for Sophia to dream her own dreams about fairies and happy things.

Leonie

Leonie's father, Bob, had died suddenly and unexpectedly, causing great distress and sadness to many who knew him. Leonie consulted me some six months after the funeral, saying that her life had suffered enormously since his death. She continued to cry uncontrollably and was not 'able to get on with her life' nor forget about her father. Many people had encouraged her to 'forget and move on' and Leonie had been endeavouring to do this with great difficulty. This difficulty was talking her into thinking she was a failure and silly and that she should have felt better by now.

I asked for permission to inquire about her father and the memories of him that Leonie cherished. I asked about the effect of the ideas of disconnecting, moving on and forgetting her father had had on Leonie. Leonie spoke of the burden she felt and the drain in energy it required to try to push his memories away. I wondered what it would be like for her to have these memories closer rather than more distant from her. What difference did Leonie think this would make? Leonie was surprised by this suggestion but spoke of how she thought it would assist her.

Our conversations then centred around the memories and recollections she had of her father, the way he had lived his life and the similarities and differences that they had appreciated in one another. I asked Leonie what she thought her father would say if he could witness her tears and sorrow over his death. Leonie was interested in this idea but somewhat puzzled by this question, so I asked her if there was anyone who might know about what her father might say about her sorrow. Leonie instantly named her father's life-long friend, Ted. She explained that Ted and her father 'knew everything about each other, and really respected each other'. I asked Leonie if she would be interested in Ted's

views on this question (i.e. what her father would say if he could witness her sorrow and tears). She was very interested as she said it would mean a lot to her to know what her dad would say to her at this time of sadness.

We invited Ted to our next session and I interviewed him about his knowledge of Leonie's father. We heard many stories of the special relationship that Bob had shared with his daughter. Ted thought that Bob would feel honoured that Leonie felt such sadness as he thought that Bob would experience her tears as an acknowledgement of what they shared together. I asked Ted about some of those times. He shared a story about Leonie and Bob regularly attending football matches together. As he was telling us this, I noticed that Leonie became very tearful. I asked her about her tears. Leonie told us that she just realised that since her father's death she had been unable to watch or attend a football game as she thought that this would be 'disrespectful' to her father.

Hearing Ted speak in this conversation helped Leonie considerably. She described how she sensed her father's presence strongly as Ted spoke. She made many decisions as a result of this meeting that contributed positively to her life – for instance she and Ted now regularly attend football matches together to honour Bob. Ted has written to me since the meeting to express the impact of the conversation on his life: 'Speaking about Bob like we did helped me to realise that I don't have to forget him. Leonie and I have a great time together now and our time together is now a very important part of my life.'

Reciprocal sharing

Re-membering conversations more directly acknowledge the valued contributions that others have made to the lives of people consulting the therapist. It is a reciprocal type of sharing. People who are identified and included in these conversations experience them as powerfully acknowledging and honouring of them also. This honouring, in turn, contributes to their lives being more richly described. Often what is discovered is that there are many similarities between the preferences, commitments, beliefs or valued ways of living between the person consulting the therapist and the person(s) whose membership is acknowledged. Through re-membering conversations, people become joined in these similarities and shared beliefs in ways that often create

further possibilities for action for everyone involved in the conversations. People feel joined in their beliefs, commitments and preferences for living. As these are discussed and elevated through the therapist's questions, they become more visible and cherished.

Summary

Memories and histories of connection become more available when people are invited to engage in re-membering conversations. People are able to link and join with significant others in their lives around shared values, commitments and preferences, in ways that powerfully contribute to the history of alternative stories. People have told me that this way of linking with the important members of their club of life has meant that they experience the presence of these significant people in their lives more vividly in their daily interactions, and that this opens up possibilities that otherwise would not have existed. Re-membering conversations can also involve deliberate decisions to exclude certain people from the membership of a person's life, people who may have contributed to the life of the problem story (see Zoe's story in chapter 10). By privileging those memberships that are deemed to be supportive of a person's wishes and ambitions in life, and by revoking the memberships of those who contribute to the life of the problem, re-membering conversations can play a significant part in the re-authoring process.

Further reading

Epston, D., Freeman, J. & Lobovits, D. 1997: 'Unlicensed co-therapists.' In Epston, D., Freeman, J. & Lobovits, D. (eds), *Playful Approaches to Serious Problems: Narrative therapy with children and their families,* chapter 9. New York: Norton.

White, M. 1988: 'Saying hullo again: The incorporation of the lost relationship in the resolution of grief.' Reprinted in White, C. & Denborough, D. (eds) 1998: *Introducing Narrative Therapy: A collection of practice-based writings.* Adelaide: Dulwich Centre Publications.

White, M. 1997: 'Re-membering.' In White, M., *Narratives of Therapists Lives,* chapter 2. Adelaide: Dulwich Centre Publications.

Chapter 10

Therapeutic documentation:
Documents, declarations, certificates, handbooks, notes from the session, videotapes, lists, pictures

As people re-author their lives and relationships, certain knowledges about the problem and the person's preferences for living become clearer. The dominant story's influence diminishes as new and preferred stories emerge. Therapeutic documentation records these preferences, knowledges and commitments so they are available for people to access at any time.

Therapeutic documents

Therapeutic documents are often written when people make important commitments or when people are ready to celebrate important achievements. Documents are written in consultation with people and contain the information they judge to be important. The therapist ascertains from the family how they would like the document to be written and what they intend doing with it. Some people have been known to carry these documents with them at all times, in their handbags or wallet, so that they are easily accessed when required.

These documents can be private or can have a wide readership,

recruiting an audience to the new and preferred meanings that are evolving for the people who are seeking assistance. They often serve as 'counter-documents' to the problem-saturated documentation of people's lives that often occurs in various institutions (schools, hospitals, welfare systems, prisons, etc.).

Documents may also include letters to and from significant people that follow on from re-membering conversations. They may record the history of all the steps that have led up to a significant unique outcome. They may describe how much of a person's life has been reclaimed from a particular problem's influence and how this has occurred. Or they may document agreements or suggestions that have been made in a therapy session.

Having a written document that records the commitments and directions that people have chosen often assists them to reclaim their lives from the influence of problems. People subjected to the voices of schizophrenia, for example, have said that they find documents particularly useful (see Brigitte, Sue, Mem & Veronika, 1997, Power to Our Journeys 1999). When faced by an attack from the voices, they read their 'document of identity'. They say this assists them to stay connected to their own hopes, skills, competencies and ways of living, and that this is very helpful.

It is difficult, in this introductory book, to illustrate the diversity of ways in which therapeutic documents can be written and used. There are infinite possibilities. I have included here just two examples, and would encourage you to experiment with your own.

Family peace document

The following document was written with the Anderson family. The family members decided to put one copy on the fridge in the kitchen and that each family member would put a copy in their bedrooms. This document was to remind them of the commitments they had made to Family Peace.

All members of the Anderson Family have agreed that fighting and bickering have been separating their family and causing problems for too long. The Andersons are interested in continuing to develop Family Peace because they all prefer it. Those members who have signed this document agree to:

Co-operation and sharing during TV watching. Each member will consult other family members and vote on the program that the majority of members are interested in watching. Those who do not get their first preference will refrain from tantrums and crying, and instead will negotiate to videotape their program for later viewing.

Sticking to the roster of chores that has been agreed upon. No discussions will be entered into by anyone about the roster until the review meeting.

Taking turns sitting in the front seat of the car. In doing this, family members understand that this decision will not always be fair. They have decided upon this course of action in the interests of gaining Family Peace.

Each person will respect an individual's item of clothing and bedroom. If a family member wishes to borrow an item of clothing or enter someone else's bedroom, they will consult the owner before doing so.

This document will be reviewed in one week's time for comment.

Signed ... (by family members)

Ivor's steps against Panic and for Happiness

Ivor wrote the following two documents with his therapist. The first document describes the Panic that was wreaking havoc in Ivor's life. The second document, entitled 'Steps for Happiness', is a counter-document. It describes the counter-plot or alternative story. These documents were written after the therapist had ensured that abuse was not a part of the context of Ivor's life.

Whereas some documents are fixed and never changed, others may become 'works in progress'. These more fluid, changing and responsive pieces allow for the recording of significant details and events in the emerging, new and preferred alternative story.

1. Ivor's knowledge about PANIC

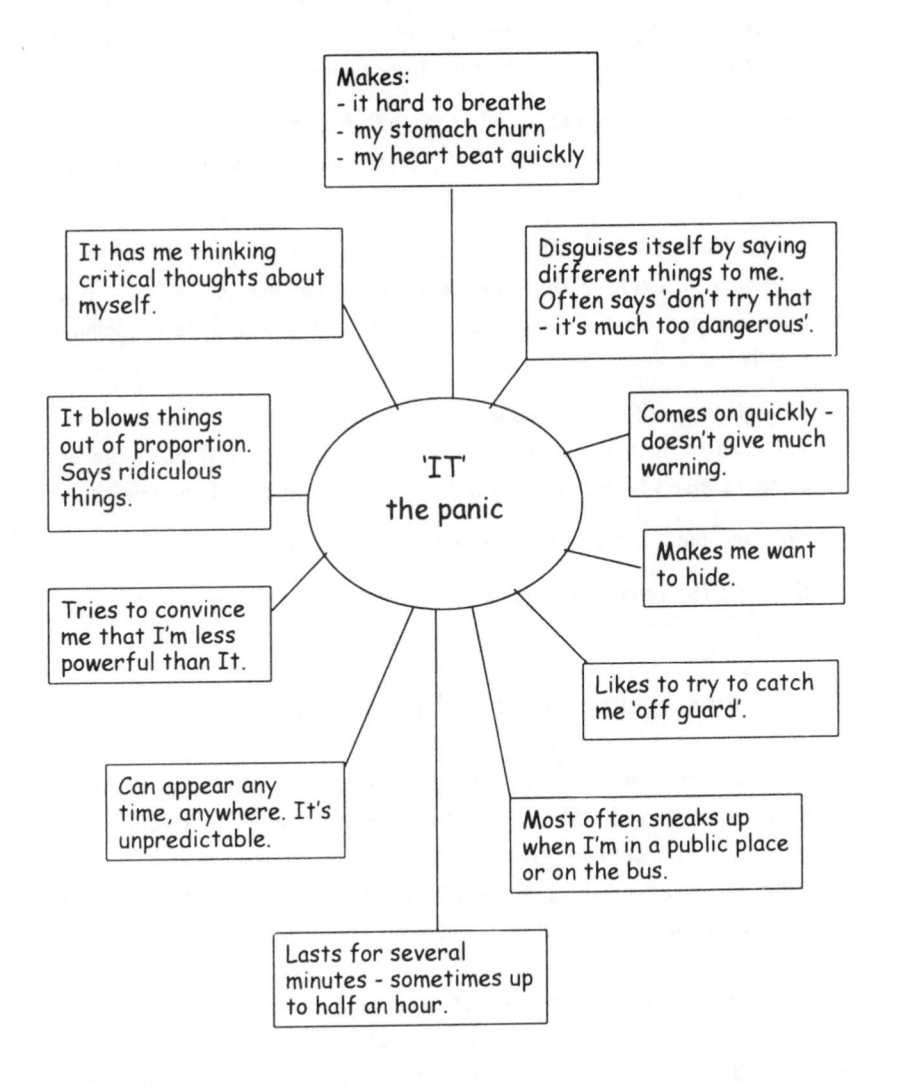

Makes:
- it hard to breathe
- my stomach churn
- my heart beat quickly

It has me thinking critical thoughts about myself.

Disguises itself by saying different things to me. Often says 'don't try that - it's much too dangerous'.

It blows things out of proportion. Says ridiculous things.

Comes on quickly - doesn't give much warning.

'IT' the panic

Makes me want to hide.

Tries to convince me that I'm less powerful than It.

Likes to try to catch me 'off guard'.

Can appear any time, anywhere. It's unpredictable.

Most often sneaks up when I'm in a public place or on the bus.

Lasts for several minutes - sometimes up to half an hour.

2. Ivor's steps against Panic

'For Happiness'

1. Deciding 'I want It out of my life'.

2. Discovering It tells lies.

3. Continuing to do things despite what It says – looking Panic 'in the eye'.

4. Exposing It and working out what It tries to tell me.

5. Remembering that I have managed to successfully challenge Panic on at least 5 different occasions.

6. Knowing about all the things I do to minimise the Panic like:

   ❖ finding something else to think about or do

   ❖ getting to a safe place

   ❖ staying around people who care for me when I know I'm feeling vulnerable

   ❖ concentrating on taking slow, deep, calm breaths

   ❖ asking myself 'Could that really happen?'

To be continued ... ...

Declarations

Declarations are similar to therapeutic documents although they tend to be used more publicly. They are written with the intention of sharing them with others. Finding witnesses to a declaration is another way to recruit an audience to the new and preferred story, but is not mandatory. Sometimes people may choose to keep their declarations to themselves. People may be invited to write a declaration stating a position, a commitment or perhaps a preference that has significance for them in the new story. Ashley said, 'The act of writing a declaration seems to make it "set in concrete" and much more real and meaningful than just saying it. I was amazed at just how many times I referred to it.'

Zoe consulted me about abuse she had been subjected to by an ordained member of the Catholic Church. It was Zoe's intention to disconnect her associations from the formal institution of the church. Zoe wrote a four-page 'Declaration of Independence' stating her position in relation to the church, her future intentions and beliefs. This document was read on several occasions to assembled audiences of supporters who were invited to witness and sign the document to show their support. Not only did this declaration provide Zoe with continued strength to reclaim her life from the effects of abuse, it also supported her in the process of claiming financial compensation for the abuse. Before meeting with the church's barrister and psychiatrist, Zoe read and re-read her declaration with the signatures of thirty-eight people who had signed it. Having the document and signatures of her supporters, she said, gave her strength to keep going with the various stages involved in pursuing her claim and with facing the Compensation Panel.

Declarations can be as simple as a one-word statement written during a session, or longer and more formal such as Zoe's. I have found that people sometimes write these declarations away from sessions and bring them proudly with them to our next meeting. Lisa told me that, one day when she was out having lunch with her friends and bulimia nervosa was forbidding her from joining them in eating, she decided: 'I'm not going to put up with this anymore. It is ruining my fun.' She went home that afternoon and designed a poster on her computer with those very words elaborately printed in large letters. She made several copies and placed them in significant places where she thought bulimia might try to ambush her. At the session we named these posters her 'Declaration for Fun and Living'. Lisa often referred to this declaration when faced with the isolation of bulimia. She showed it to a close friend who was honoured to be included in Lisa's life in this way. Lisa found this declaration extremely sustaining and told me that writing it, reading it and sharing it with her friend was a very important turning point in reclaiming her life.

Certificates

Certificates can be drawn up and signed to commemorate significant events and turning points. Certificates help to celebrate the new story that

emerges and to commemorate how the person has managed to overcome the problem to regain their life from its influence.

The title for the certificate often comes from the names given to the problem and the alternative story during the course of therapy. It may be a certificate to commemorate a skill, personal quality, desire, hope, commitment, action, statement, competence or preference that has been discovered and richly described in the new story. It could be a certificate for bravery, courage, intelligence, temper taming and fear catching, confidence, trust or self-belief. The certificate could be phrased using the (now obsolete) problem name: for example:

- An escape from *Self-Doubt*

- Breaking the grip of *Guilt*

- Freedom from a *Drug lifestyle*

- Beating *Dishonesty*

- Breaking from *Violence*

In each example the word in italics can be substituted for the name given to the problem. Alternatively, the certificate might name and commemorate the alternative story. For example:

- Reclaiming happiness and sparkle

- Getting to know patience

- Navigating the journey of courage

- Five hard-won wisdoms

- Standing in solidarity

- Celebrating connectedness

I sent Freiya the following certificate when she had successfully banished 'the habits' to the sun and 'stuck to the path of getting things done'.

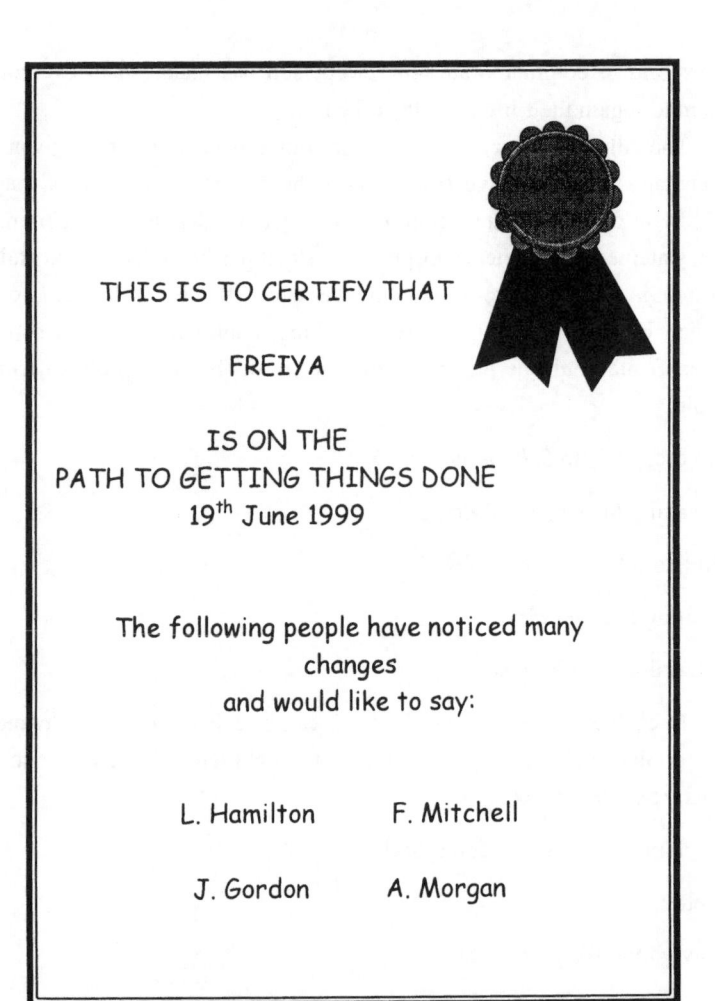

THIS IS TO CERTIFY THAT

FREIYA

IS ON THE
PATH TO GETTING THINGS DONE
19th June 1999

The following people have noticed many
changes
and would like to say:

L. Hamilton   F. Mitchell

J. Gordon   A. Morgan

Alirra received the following certificate when 'the headaches' were no longer in her life. A special ceremony was conducted and a formal presentation of the certificate was made to Alirra in the presence of her parents, two teachers, a friend and myself. The commemorative chocolate cake that was prepared for the celebration was delicious (see chapter 12 for a further description of the celebration).

The possibilities for such certificates are endless.

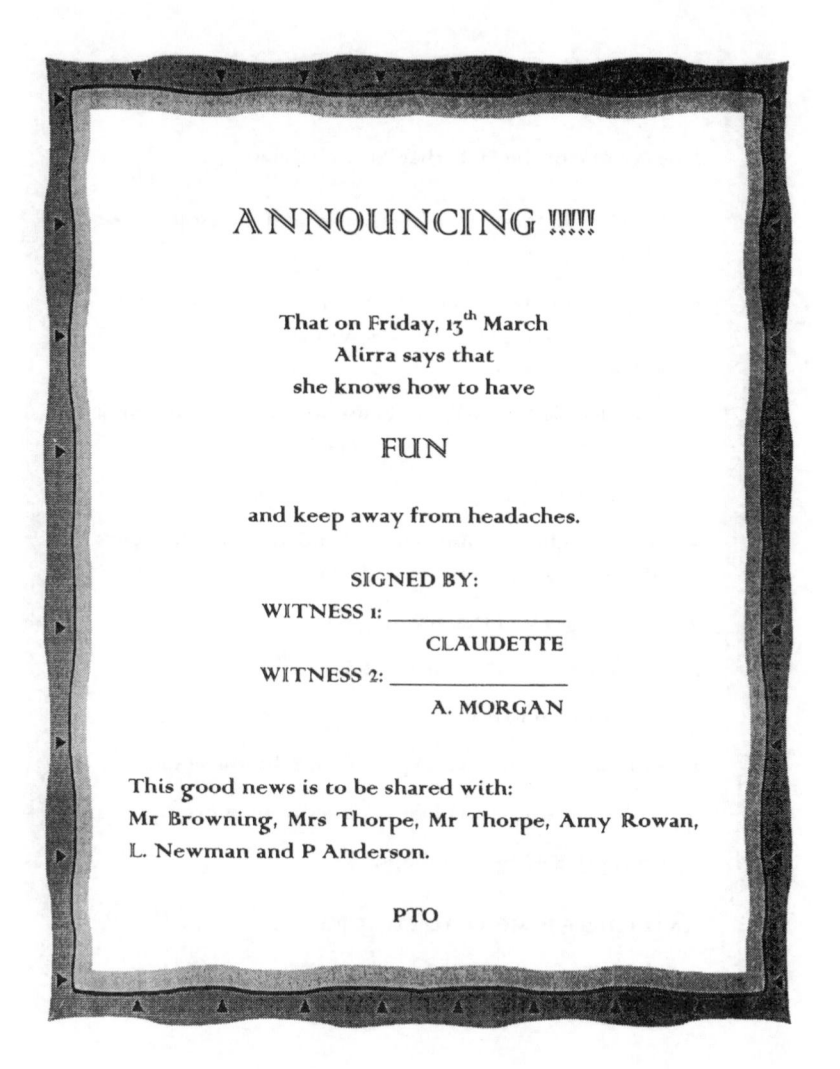

ANNOUNCING !!!!!

That on Friday, 13th March
Alirra says that
she knows how to have

FUN

and keep away from headaches.

SIGNED BY:
WITNESS 1: _____
CLAUDETTE

WITNESS 2: _____
A. MORGAN

This good news is to be shared with:
Mr Browning, Mrs Thorpe, Mr Thorpe, Amy Rowan,
L. Newman and P Anderson.

PTO

This is some of the FUN that Alirra has had:

➤ Staying at Amy Rowan's house and playing 'Spice Girls'.

➤ Staying up late and not going to sleep at Amy's place, telling ghost stories, and having a midnight snack.

➤ Amy has been to Alirra's house to stay and did a play together.

➤ Rollerskating party.

➤ Went to Ellie's house twice, bumped down the stairs on sleeping bags, and swam in the pool.

➤ Watching TV in the morning.

➤ Having McDonald's for breakfast.

➤ Going to Canberra.

➤ Swimming in the Hyatt pool with Sally for hours.

➤ Watching Hot-air Balloons at 6.30 in the morning.

➤ Going to Teddy Bear shops.

AND THERE IS MORE TO COME !!!!! ......>......

Handbooks

Handbooks are another way to formally record people's knowledges and expertise. Some of the titles of handbooks that I recall have proved helpful have included:

- *How to Escape from Fears and Worry*

- *What Children Know about Separation and Divorce*

- *Kid's Temper Tamer Handbook: How to Cool Off and Be Cool*

These handbooks collect the stories of those with experience of these issues. They contain the person's ideas, thoughts and abilities in counteracting a problem's motives and ways. People newer to a problem's ways can have access to the handbooks of others, via their therapist, and can find the knowledge of others sustaining of them in their journey. Reading the stories of others may encourage them to add their experiences and ideas to an existing handbook, or alternatively to write their own handbook, telling their story in a different way.

In such handbooks, people may record milestones on their journey or write cumulative statements of their progressions along the way. The therapist might encourage them to make additions to the handbook when unique outcomes emerge, as a way of confirming and documenting the change and the new story based on their strengths and competencies. When handbooks are lent to others, this is not with the intention that they be used as expert guidance. They are not recipes for others. Instead, the intention is to share knowledges and celebrate successes. The helpfulness of handbooks lies just as much in the reading of them as in the writing of them.

Some handbooks become collaborative, public documents where every reader is invited to contribute their expertise and add their discoveries to those previously recorded. Space in this publication does not permit the printing of such a handbook. However, the reading list will assist readers to pursue this area further.

Notes from the session and video or audiotapes

During consultations, the therapist may take written notes to keep track of the important things that are being said and to help them guide the direction of the conversation. For example, I usually record unique outcomes and particular phrases or expressions used by people to describe the alternative story (i.e. things standing outside of the problem-saturated story). The therapist always asks the family for permission to take notes during the session, and most narrative therapists consider these notes to be the property of the family. When I am seeking permission to take notes, I explain that I will only record the words of family members (not my words), that I will tell them what I am writing down and that I will check the accuracy of what I am writing with them. I explain that the notes belong to them and that they are welcome to take them at the end of the session. I sometimes ask for permission to keep a copy, explaining my intentions or thoughts about doing so.

Families have told me that they have found these notes useful to refer to between sessions. Families have said that to see their words in writing reminds them of the conversation and the ideas that arose during it. They comment on how the notes assist them to shift from the ideas that are associated with their perceptions of the problem to ideas about their lives that fit with the commitments and preferences that have been more richly described in the therapeutic conversation.

Therapists who have access to videotaping or audiotaping facilities may offer to record the conversation for the family. Again most narrative therapists would consider these tapes to be the property of the family and would clearly discuss the purposes of such recordings at the outset. Some families like to keep copies of these recordings, whilst others return them at the following session to be taped over with their next conversation. Some family members like to review the tapes between sessions or perhaps show it to someone who was absent from a particular session. If tapes are kept over the course of several meetings, they become an interesting historical record of the developments that occur. These tapes can also be useful when families experience a 'setback'. Viewing or listening to previous helpful conversations can be sustaining and can counteract the disillusionment that people are vulnerable to at these times.

Lists

Lists can be a quick and easy way to record aspects of conversations which make it possible to keep track of experiences. Lists may be compiled to record significant developments, ideas and contributions. These lists can be added to as new discoveries are made. Martin used a list to record the steps he had taken in his 'Courage and Bravery project'. Each time we met, he added more items to the list until they numbered fifty – the number of steps he predicted would be necessary to complete the project.

When significant achievements are listed and read back to people, they become more 'real' and clearer to them. Lists also assist people to revisit their knowledges and skills and to continuously record their developments.

Ben and his therapist, Jill, discussed the effect that Rushing was having on his schoolwork. Ben was interested in reclaiming his learning from these negative effects. Together he and Jill listed the things that helped him to go forward and to stand aside from Rushing, and what it was that took him back into Rushing. Ben attached this list to the front of his workbooks, and some of his classmates were so impressed with Ben's list that they wanted copies.

Ben's list

What helps me go forward:	What takes me back:
Slowing down	Rushing
Having time to think	Not thinking
Blocking out distractions	Guessing
Being sensible	Being distracted
Listening	Messy work
Keep talking to a minimum	Talking
Slowing down means neat work	Not listening
Take time to listen to the sounds of the letters	Being silly

A discussion of the therapy that Ben was involved in with Jill is detailed in Huntley 1999.

Pictures

Pictures can also assist people to stay connected to an emerging alternative story. These pictures can be either drawn or collected from other sources, for example, magazines, books, posters, photographs.

When I meet with children I find that they often like to draw as we are talking. These drawings become part of the documentation of the therapy and make a significant contribution to sustaining the positive developments that occur. For example, after I had checked out that abuse was not a part of the context of Allyssa's life, it was the use of pictures that proved influential in reducing the degree of Fear which she was experiencing. Allyssa drew a series of pictures representing the size of the Fear in relation to her size, and pictures that illustrated the ways in which she was getting the Fear out of her life. These pictures formed a story of Allyssa's abilities to regain her life from the influence of Fear.

This is not uncommon. I have noticed that when I engage in re-authoring conversations with children, their drawings often feature events or aspects of the new story rather than aspects that place the focus on the problem-saturated story. Sometimes their drawings can predict future developments. These drawings of the future can act as a prophecy and provide some motivation, support and encouragement to children to reach the new destinations they aspire to. Sometimes children choose to draw pictures that are seemingly unrelated to the therapeutic conversation. On these occasions they have told me that this does not matter because when they look at the picture it reminds them of the details of our conversation. Often children choose to take their drawings home and share them with others. In this way, the drawings become part of a retelling of the conversation and recruit an important audience to developments in the child's life.

Pictures can also have symbolic meaning. Theshara consulted me about the effects of Depression on her life. Throughout these consultations she brought to the session a greeting card or picture that had particular meaning and significance to her. Upon reflection, she concluded that over the course of our meetings her choice of cards and pictures was changing. The cards and pictures were gaining in colour and hope – in parallel with events that were occurring in her own life. These symbols offered us a starting place for our conversations as

we explored the meanings she ascribed to them. Theshara kept these pictures and cards in a diary to record her journey away from Depression. She added comments next to these symbols and this assisted her to stay connected to her hopes for happiness. Theshara told me that the symbols were far more helpful to her than the written word. She explained that one of Depression's tactics was to prevent her from reading – it often tried to distract her when she attempted to do so. These pictures become another of Theshara's tools for regaining happiness.

Summary

This chapter has explored a range of different ways of documenting therapeutic conversations: documents, declarations, certificates, handbooks, notes from the session, audio and videotapes, lists, and pictures. I have not described here the ways in which music and song can also be used as forms of therapeutic documentation. Nor have I explored the ways in which community arts projects can act as collective forms of documentation of preferred alternative community stories (Stiles 1999). The possibilities are endless. All of these mediums can be used as resources to assist in the documentation and further exploration of alternative stories. Whereas the intricacies of a conversation can so easily be forgotten, therapeutic documents can be referred to over and over again. Each reading (or playing or drawing) can act as a retelling of the alternative story, and this in turn contributes to new possibilities.

Further reading

Epston, D., Freeman, J. & Lobovits, D. 1997: 'Publishing the news.' In Epston, D., Freeman, J. & Lobovits, D. (eds), *Playful Approaches to Serious Problems: Narrative therapy with children and their families,* chapter 7. New York: Norton.

Chapter 11

Therapeutic letters

Within narrative practices, letters are used in variety of ways to assist families. David Epston and Michael White (1990) have introduced a number of different sorts of therapeutic letters including:

- letters as summary of the session

- letters of invitation and to build relationships

- letters of redundancy

- letters of reference

There are many pieces that have been written on the use of letters in narrative therapy (see further reading list) so in this chapter I will only provide a short description of each of these different types of letters.

Before letters are sent

Before the therapist sends a letter, they always consult the family about this idea. They ask the family members if they would be interested in receiving a letter and, if so, they inquire as to the reasons for this interest. The therapist might explain some of the possibilities as to the content of the letter and ask the family members which of the possibilities appeals to them. Issues of confidentiality are important to consider at this time, so the therapist needs to

ascertain how the letter should be addressed. Therapists can prepare the family for receiving a letter by asking them what they think they would be likely to do with the letter – would they read it just once or more often? where would they keep it? – and to predict its likely effects. The therapist can also explain that he or she will be interested, at the next meeting, in hearing the family's comments about the letter and about the effects of receiving it. In this way, the therapist can set a context whereby the family members feel comfortable to suggest changes, deletions and additions to the letter and can ask them for their ideas about which parts of the present conversation they think would be important to include in the next letter.

Letters as summary

From time to time the therapist will write to the people consulting them, providing a summary of the conversations they have shared. These letters may contain any of the following:

- some of the main ideas or thoughts that emerged during the conversations

- questions that the therapist has wondered about since the conversation

- some reflections from the therapist about the conversation

- documentation of some of the unique outcomes that were discovered during the session

- requests for clarification about some part of the conversation that the therapist would like to be clearer about

- aspects of the conversation that were not fully explored during the session that may be of interest to the person receiving the letter

When writing these letters, the therapist is careful to use the language and words that were spoken during the session. Therapeutic letters contain the names the family has given to the dominant and alternative stories, and the language of externalising conversations and questions. Often the notes that therapists make during a conversation enable them to write letters that include the exact phrasing and expressions that were helpful to the people concerned.

Therapeutic letters, which vary in length, content and form, become an extension of the therapy session. Therapists develop their own personal style of writing these letters. Receiving feedback from the people to whom the letters are written plays a large part in this process.

The following letter was written to Penny after a conversation about the hostile voices of schizophrenia. The letter contains summaries of the things that Penny told the therapist, some questions posed by the therapist, and direct quotations from the session itself. The letter moves between past, present and future time frames and details the names of the problem (the hostile voices) and the emerging alternative story (the upper hand), while focusing predominantly on the alternative story. This emphasis is intentional. It is assumed that documenting the alternative story will assist Penny to stay more connected to it and that this will contribute to her future actions being shaped positively by it.

Dear Penny,

I thought I'd write you this letter after we met on Tuesday because there were so many things you told me that caught my attention and that I've since been curious about.

You described how 'the hostile voices' were quieter this past week and that you had managed to have 'the upper hand' in most instances. I was wondering more about your 'upper hand' and asked you if you had noticed it before. You told me that you thought that you must have been training it over the past few months but that this was the first time that you had used it. I was wondering more about that training and how you did that? It sounded as though all the practice you did with your 'upper hand' was rewarding as you said that the 'hostile voices' only tried to retaliate when you had ideas of going to meet Sally at the bus stop. Even then though, your 'upper hand' silenced the hostile voices and you managed to go on your outing.

I was wondering what it has been like for you to do all this? What personal strengths or qualities did you use? I was wondering also if Sally knew what you were up against in meeting her that day? If she did, what would she say it took?

We also talked about the freedom and fun you had got back over the past few weeks. You said that even if the voices insisted on whispering to you that 'at least they didn't boom at me like they usually do'. You spoke of your increased freedom to be in the garden, to have fun watching TV and making

phone calls, and the freedom to care for yourself more.

I was wondering if there was anyone who would have predicted that you would get back your fun and freedom from the hostile voices and reclaim your fun and freedom in the ways that you have done? Maybe you could tell me next time we meet.

There are lots of questions in this letter. Some of them might be interesting to you and others not – we can talk about them next time if you wish or anything else that is important to you. I'll look forward to hearing about your trip to the city and I'd love to see that photo, if you remember! Kind Regards, Alice

Many people have told me that receiving a letter such as the one above can be very helpful. They have found the written word sustaining as it reminds them of the conversation shared. Letters that summarise a conversation and contain some further questions also assist people to stay connected to the emerging alternative story that is co-authored in narrative meetings. When people are more connected to the preferred stories of their lives, they are more likely to continue to be able to get free from the influence of the problem.

After Trish had received a similar sort of letter to the one sent to Penny, she said: 'I couldn't believe you would spend the time to write to me. It made me feel so much stronger in relation to Anxiety to know that someone else was with me in the fight. I read it so many times during the week – it really helped to bring Anxiety out of the shadows. I noticed I could fight it a bit more'.

Brief letters

Brief letters that contain perhaps only one or two questions or sentences can also make a positive contribution to people's lives.

I wrote this short note to Samuel after a session in which he told me about his intentions to apply for a job in the newspaper. Samuel was interested in reclaiming his interest in music and intended to pursue work in this area for the first time in twelve years. An abusive incident had resulted in him being totally disconnected from his musical talents and had prevented him from even looking in the relevant section of the newspaper for several years. Samuel and I had discussed the steps leading to this breakthrough and had celebrated them in

our conversation together. I sent him this note:

> Samuel,
>
> *Since we talked I couldn't stop wondering who was 'standing with you', supporting you when you decided to buy that first newspaper and begin to look in the music section. Were you totally alone or was there someone 'behind' you?*
>
> *Alice*

This short letter assisted Samuel to consider those people who had assisted him along the path of reclaiming music in his life (see chapter 9, Remembering conversations). He later said that having these people more in his consciousness at the time of taking these important steps gave him more determination to continue than he might otherwise have had.

Letters of summary can take many creative forms. Amy, a six-year-old girl, was particularly interested in the pop group The Spice Girls. I sent Amy a Spice Girls sticker that was stuck on a piece of paper with a large speech bubble containing an appropriate question from Scary Spice, Amy's favourite character. Sometimes it can be helpful to send drawings or pictures to people. Freiya was 'on the road to getting things done' and expressed her immense satisfaction in her ability to stick to this path. One day, when reading a magazine, I found a beautiful picture of a series of paths through dense bushland and forest. I sent it to Freiya and wrote the following: 'This picture reminded me of the path that you told me you had chosen. I was wondering how you chose it from all the other ones? How did you know it would suit you?'

Letters of invitation and letters to build relationships

Letters can also be useful in inviting people to attend meetings with the therapist and various family members. The reasons for such an invitation are made clear to the people who are being invited, and an opportunity is made for them to respond to the invitation.

Lauren received this letter from me:

> Dear Lauren,
>
> *I have spoken to your mum and she's told me about what's going on at*

the moment. I've been thinking about you and wondered if it would help to come and have a chat sometime. I've met your sister before and would like to get to know you too. What do you think?
From Mrs Morgan

Other people who are significant in the life of the person consulting the therapist, but who are not family members, can also be invited to attend sessions.

Dear Mardie,

As you know, Michele and I have met a few times to discuss some things that are important to her. The other day she told me that you had made a comment about something she had done at school when she was younger that Michele was very curious about. Michele and I are interested in hearing some more about what you know about Michele's abilities at school and we were wondering if you would be able to meet with us? I would ask you a few questions, if that is ok, so that Michele can hear about that part of her life. I hope you are interested in joining in this project and look forward to meeting you.

Best wishes, Alice Morgan

Letters of invitation can also help to introduce people to the therapist, and establish the beginnings of a relationship prior to direct conversation. This can assist people with their decision to consult a therapist about a particular difficulty.

Loretta Perry wrote a series of letters to a young boy, Finn, who had not spoken in his family for some time. The first letter of a series is included below. At the time that Loretta sent it, Finn had not attended any therapy sessions. Loretta had spoken to Josie, Finn's caretaker, who provided some ideas to assist Loretta with the letter. This letter contains invitations, therapeutic comments and questions and it served to develop a connection between Loretta and Finn. Loretta wrote seven further letters before she received a response from Finn. This is an example of how letters can be used to build connections to people when simply turning up to a therapy appointment is not an option for them. (All the letters and a discussion of the therapy are detailed in Perry 1999.)

Dear Finn,

I was disappointed that our first appointment fell through, so I thought

I'd write. I've been told by Josie that you're on retreat – I hear the retreat's been going seven months. Some time ago I watched a show on television and was fascinated to learn about individuals, perhaps like yourself, who commit to and join what they call 'Orders'. Orders invite vows of silence and promises from the people, sometimes forever – have you heard about this? Of course the interviewer couldn't talk to the people on retreat, so they had to ask questions of their family members, or of their old friends if they didn't have any family people around. None of the people on retreat seemed to have made any new friends since the vows of silence. The interviewer asked them some questions about the silence that had taken them over – questions like: Did silence have to work hard and for a long time before it won you over? Or did silence convince you to commit to it overnight? Does silence on the outside mean silence on the inside? And does a commitment to forever mean forever? The interviewer asked things like that.

Finn, I was wondering whether there were any similarities between the commitment you've made to silence and the ideas put forward in the show. The show grabbed my attention, and left me wanting to know more about people that silence calls upon. You see, because of the time constraint there were some things left unsaid, particularly in relation to one young woman – she wasn't as young as you though. But, all in all, the show got me thinking.

I'd really love to meet you but fully understand if the vows you've taken prevent this from happening. If the commitment to silence doesn't want you to come back to a speaking world just yet, could an old friend of yours, or someone from your family, come in your place, just like in the television show ...?

Loretta

PS: How do you get to know what's going on in the world outside your retreat? Do you send your eyes and ears outside while you stay indoors?

Letters of redundancy

These letters may be written to someone who is seeking to make redundant some job or role they may have once fulfilled during the time they

were under the influence of a particular problem. Some problems invite parents to take particular roles that assist their child during the time they are faced with the difficulty. As the child makes steps away from the problem's influence, this role may be no longer required. This was the situation with Allyssa. Fears had been preventing her from sleeping in her bedroom alone. She was continually tired and this made it difficult for her to remember to bring things to school. It also meant that she was often 'disorganised' and 'forgetful'.

After checking out that abuse was not a contributing factor, we explored the relationship between Allyssa and her mother, Pam. Pam supported Allyssa as she shrunk the Fear, by offering to remind her of the items she needed to take to school and agreeing to make special trips to school if she forgot certain necessary items, for example, music equipment or sports clothes. Pam looked forward to returning to the times when Allyssa was able to do this for herself.

Allyssa was successful in getting Fear out of her life and began to sleep soundly in her bedroom. As she regained her energy she began to notice that she didn't need her mum to do all the tasks for her that she had taken on. We wrote Pam this letter with the good news.

Dear Pam,

Today Allyssa and I have talked about some of the changes she has noticed since she has got her life back from Fears. Allyssa told me that now she can sleep better, she has found that she is more 'in control of her life' and that she can 'remember things now'. Allyssa is very pleased about this and her ability to organise her own things. When I asked her what you would think, Allyssa thought you would be excited too. Allyssa announced today that this means 'I don't need my mum to do it anymore, because I know that I can do it now'. I guess that means that you won't need to worry about the reminders and the organising job you had and will have some more time on your hands. How is that for you? I remember once you telling me you couldn't wait for this day to come, so I'll look forward to hearing what you do with it!

Allyssa also said that she wanted to thank you a lot for what you did to keep her life going as she shrunk Fear and she has made some plans for how to do this. I won't spoil the surprise!

Regards, Alice Morgan

Letters of reference

These letters are usually written 'To whom it may concern' and contain accounts of a person's developing identity, one that is not defined by the problem that has been influencing their lives. The therapist writes this type of letter in consultation with the person and often multiple copies are made for wide distribution. These letters can be particularly helpful in situations where a problem has invited a certain 'reputation' into the person's life. These negative reputations can be difficult to shift, so a letter such as this may assist those around the person to begin to entertain a new and more positive reputation. These letters contribute to shifting the accounts of the person that were once problem-saturated to new, more positive ones.

Shaun was regaining his life from Trouble. His family and school were concerned about the effect that Trouble was having on him. As Shaun regained his life from the problem, the following letter of reference was written. Shaun requested fifteen copies be made and sent to 'key' people like his teachers, his friends and members of his family.

To Whom It May Concern:

As you know, Shaun has been regaining his life from Trouble for several months now. I have been meeting with Shaun to discuss his achievements and thought you may like to be kept up to date on the following:

- It is now 33 days since Shaun was required to attend a detention.

- Shaun has completed and submitted all the work that is due and is currently up to date on all assignments.

- Shaun has been having victories over Lying.

- Shaun thinks that his attitude to study is more positive and that he wants to stay at school.

- Shaun intends to 'own up to' the graffiti he wrote and offer to clean it off the walls.

Although it is still early days, Shaun intends to continue to challenge

Trouble's ways and continue with these developments.

I am writing you this note to invite you to collect further evidence of Shaun's life moving away from Trouble and to inform you that these achievements may require you to treat Shaun somewhat differently than the ways of the past.

What do you think? I would be happy to hear from any of you that may have further ideas or comments to make.

Best wishes
Alice Morgan

Summary

Within narrative practices, therapeutic letter writing often plays a significant part. In some circumstances, the entire therapy can occur through letters (e.g. where direct conversation is impossible). Letter writing can also be particularly significant in situations where people are unsure as to whether they wish to talk to a therapist (i.e. in involuntary situations). In these situations letters can provide a less threatening opening to a relationship than talking face-to-face. In other situations, letters act as a parallel process to actual conversation, contributing to the thickening of alternative stories and providing reflections that can be referred to at any time.

Further reading

Epston, D. 1998: 'Expanding the conversation.' In Epston, D., *Catching Up With David Epston: A collection of narrative practice-based papers published between 1991 & 1996*. Adelaide: Dulwich Centre Publications.

White, M. & Epston, D. 1990: *Narrative Means to Therapeutic Ends* (especially chapters 3 & 4). New York: Norton.

Chapter 12

Rituals and celebrations

Rituals and celebrations mark celebrate significant steps in the journey away from a problem story to a new and preferred version of life. It is difficult to write generally about rituals and ceremonies as they are as varied as the people who are involved in them. Celebrations can be formal or informal, and can take place with or without the presence of the therapist. In this section, I describe three ceremonies that I have participated in to give some sense of the possibilities.

Sonia's ritual of membership

Sonia and I planned a ceremony to elevate and privilege three relationships that were significant to her and to formally relinquish two other relationships. This idea arose from a re-membering conversation (see chapter 9) that had occurred during one of our sessions. I had inquired about who else would know of Sonia's strength and courage and of the commitment she had made to a future of 'self-belief and nurturance'. I had also asked about the people who would support, or who were currently supporting, this new direction for her life. Sonia had been disconnected from this commitment to self-belief and nurturance for much of her twenty-four years, and it had been continuously discouraged by some members of her biological family.

Sonia told me that there were three very important people in her life who supported her and encouraged her commitment to self-belief and nurturance – a teacher she had in her final year of school (Fiona), a close friend (Dianne), and her 'adopted mother' (Sadie). I invited Fiona, Dianne and Sadie to a celebration and explained its intention: to honour their contribution to Sonia's life. At the ceremony, Sonia and I read some prepared statements to Fiona, Dianne and Sadie and presented them all with Honorary Life Membership Certificates to Sonia's life. I interviewed Sonia about the significance of this to her whilst the three women listened. I then asked Fiona, Dianne and Sadie a series of questions about the contribution that Sonia had made to their lives. In this way, the reciprocal nature of their relationships was honoured and acknowledged. At this ceremony we also read prepared statements that announced the cessation of two abusive relationships that Sonia no longer wished to have in her life. The ceremony concluded with hugs, champagne and much laughter.

Alirra's ceremony of fun

Alirra had been successful in 'getting back fun and confidence' from the influence of Headaches. One day, I asked Alirra if she thought we should plan a celebration of her achievements. Alirra was delighted with the suggestion and wanted to invite some people to join us in this. The next two sessions were spent making plans. Alirra chose to invite the people who had made significant contributions to the 'getting back fun and confidence' project – her mother and father, her current teacher, her teacher from the previous year, her friend and myself. Together we made the invitations and planned the agenda for the event.

At this celebration, each participant had the opportunity to speak and reflect on Alirra's achievements and contributions. Alirra asked me to speak on her behalf about the contributions that all those who were present had made. A presentation to Alirra of a certificate to commemorate 'getting back fun and confidence' (see chapter 10) was made in the presence of her invited guests. Members of the meeting signed the certificate as witnesses. Her mother gave Alirra a present and had baked a special chocolate cake. This was decorated with balloons (a symbol of fun that Alirra and I had often spoken about) with the words 'Alirra: strong, confident, caring, determined, courage' written in

icing. These words came from conversations that Alirra, her mother and myself had shared about the personal qualities Alirra possessed that assisted her with getting back fun and confidence.

A ritual of declaration

Zoe and I planned a ritual to celebrate and publicly acknowledge her 'Declaration of Independence' (see Declarations in chapter 10). At this ritual we used the four stages of the outsider-witness group process, described in chapter 14. The formal part of the evening began after dinner. Zoe lit two candles for her two children who were overseas at the time of the meeting, and who had sent their support for the evening. The event was audiotaped and sent to them.

Family members who were invited to the event first witnessed an interview between myself and Zoe. After I had interviewed Zoe, I then interviewed the invited members about what they had heard. I invited them to reflect on the conversation they had witnessed and to comment on those aspects that particularly caught their attention. Zoe was an audience to this conversation. Zoe then had the opportunity to comment on these reflections and read her 'Declaration of Independence' to all assembled. The fourth part of the evening gave everyone the opportunity to ask me questions about why I had asked the questions I had, and about my ideas or thinking. We concluded by all signing the declaration and listening to 'What a Wonderful World' sung by Louis Armstrong Junior.

Summary

The possibilities for the use of ritual and celebration within narrative work are unlimited. The timing, scope and content of rituals are determined through a collaborative process between therapists and the people consulting them. In each circumstance, considerations are made in relation to what would be the appropriate audience and setting for the ritual, and how it could be structured in a way to most powerfully acknowledge all that has been experienced. Rituals do not necessarily have to involve celebration. Powerful

rituals of loss, grieving and moving on may also be a part of a therapeutic journey. In considering the structuring of rituals, therapists usually consider the principles that inform re-authoring conversations. Care is taken to ensure that rituals do not focus solely on the problematic story and that alternative stories are performed in appropriate settings in front of especially selected audiences. The telling and performance of alternative stories in these settings can be transformative.

Chapter 13

Expanding the conversation:
Co-research, leagues, networks, committees, groups and teams

Those people who have experience with problems, either in the present or in the past, hold special knowledges, skills, competencies and expertise that can assist others in similar situations. They have particular expertise and wisdom about, for example, the ways that particular problems operate, the ways in which problems speak, the likes and dislikes of particular problems, and the ways they have found to counteract or change their relationship with these problems.

For example, Barry, through his relationship with 'substance abuse', has special knowledges and understandings about this problem and how he managed to reclaim his life from its effects. He holds understandings about how substance abuse invites itself into people's lives, how it speaks and operates, and how he changed his relationship with substances from an 'abusive' to a more 'harmonious' one. These words were chosen by Barry to describe the changes in his relationship to substance use. These knowledges that Barry has acquired have the potential to assist and support others who are interested in reclaiming their lives from drug problems.

Imagine what it would be like to collect and record Barry's special knowledges and for these to be accessible to other people. Imagine a library of understandings about 'the voice of substance abuse' or documents that record

ways to break from the effects of certain substances on one's life. Narrative therapists assume that access to these special knowledges can further reduce the influence of such problems in the lives of those affected by them and contribute to significant shifts in understandings about ways to counteract them.

Sometimes the process of unearthing and recording people's insider knowledges is called 'consulting your consultants', or 'co-research'. It involves the documentation of people's knowledges and skills about problems and ways of addressing them, so that this knowledge can be distributed to others. This distribution of knowledge often happens through the written word. For example, documents or therapeutic letters may be circulated (with permission) between people who are struggling with similar issues.

Many narrative therapists try to find other ways to assist people to access the special knowledges and understandings held by others. Establishing and consulting leagues, committees, teams, groups and networks constitute one way this can be done. These leagues are groups of people interested in sharing their insider-knowledges with others. They bring together and circulate the voices of people who are involved in a similar struggle. In this way, it is their voices on these matters that are privileged, rather than the voices of therapists.

There are a number of ways that people have made hard-won insider-knowledges more accessible to others. These range from small-scale, local projects to large-scale, international ventures. For example, teams or networks have been established by small groups of narrative therapists and the persons consulting them. These teams or networks document and record information in the form a file or collection/resource for other people to consult. People are invited to join these groups, leagues, networks or teams that are active in standing against certain problems, and to contribute to their activities and events.

Some therapists have established books/handbooks (see chapter 10) written by the people consulting them on topics such as 'Fear Catchers', 'Monster Taming' or 'Surviving Self-abuse and Scratching'. These handbooks document the stories of those whose lives have been affected by such problems, and include rich descriptions of ways in which they have resisted the influence of the problem in their lives.

Some of these networks and leagues have a relatively recent history, whilst others have been established for some time. The Anti-Anorexia/Bulimia League has been collecting and documenting knowledges about anorexia and

bulimia nervosa for several years, and now its archives are collected in Australia, New Zealand, the United States of America and Canada. Not only do these leagues circulate many letters that have been written to undermine the voices of anorexia nervosa and bulimia nervosa, but also some members speak out publicly about a range of issues including the effects that certain images of women in the media have on women's lives.

Teaming up against a problem

The idea of having a 'Team' to assist persons to stand against the effects of a problem evokes many possibilities. To this end, therapists are often interested in opening a conversation in which other people are identified who could stand with and support the person or family experiencing the difficulty.

Sophia (aged six years) consulted me about some 'bad dreams' that had crept into her sleep and frightened her. I ascertained that abuse was not a part of this context and was then interested in exploring with Sophia ways of reducing the occurrence of these 'bad dreams'.

Sophia told me that the nightmares had lots of nasty animals on 'their side' and that she felt very powerless in their presence. I was interested in discovering from Sophia the people she thought might be on 'her side' against the bad dreams; who she thought would disapprove of what the bad dreams were up to, and, like Sophia, would want them to stay out of her sleep. I asked Sophia what she thought would happen if we got these people together on a team. What did she think would happen to the 'bad dreams' if she had more people on 'her side'? Sophia thought the team would keep her safe from the 'bad dreams' and that it would be 'good'. I asked her to name the people she knew would be on her side.

Instantly she named her mother, father, and grandmother. Further questioning led to Sophia identifying Fluffy, her toy cat, who was very important to her. Sophia explained that Fluffy slept with her and was the first to see the bad dreams in the night. A baby doll was present during this conversation and I asked Sophia whether the baby would also be on her side against the bad dreams. Sophia rather indignantly replied 'But she's only one years old!' I asked the ages of the other members of her team. We recorded them in list form on the whiteboard, and discovered that between all the team

members there was one hundred and ninety-seven years and four months of experience. Sophia confidently assured me that the 'bad dreams' did not have a hope now. We contacted all the members of the Team by phone, in person or by letter, and asked them if they would be interested in joining Sophia's 'Team Against the Bad Dreams'. They all enthusiastically agreed and certain 'jobs' were given to each of them to perform. Establishing this team during these conversations was a turning point for Sophia and contributed greatly to her reclaiming 'fairy' dreams and 'happy' dreams.

Re-membering conversations

Discussion of re-membering conversations was provided in chapter 9. I mention their significance again in this section to alert readers' attention to their potential in the 'audiencing' aspects of narrative therapy. Re-membering conversations are another way of engaging an audience to witness a person's achievements, and to witness an account of what is reflected in these achievements – special abilities, competencies, knowledges, and preferences about ways of living.

It is often possible to invite the person(s) identified through re-membering conversations to attend a session. The therapist can then interview these significant people, in the presence of the person who has come for counselling, about their thoughts, and reflections about this person. If the potential audience people are not available to attend such a session, the therapist may, with consent, phone or write to them (by letter, fax or email) and ask them about any impressions they might have of their friend's/colleague's/ acquaintance's life.

Summary

Problems often contribute to isolation, loneliness and dislocation. They also often contribute to circumstances that dishonour people's unique knowledges and know-how. Finding ways to link together people who have experienced similar difficulties, and creating processes through which these

people can share and build upon each others' skills of living is a significant part of the work of therapists engaged with narrative practices. By focussing on the linking of people's lives with those of others in helpful ways, and in creating avenues by which insider-knowledges can be shared, therapists can play an influential but de-centred role in the lives of those who consult with them.

Through the use of outsider-witness groups, leagues, networks, committees, teams, and through re-membering conversations, people's lives become linked with others in ways that more richly describe alternative stories. Sometimes this contributes to the linking of just two or three lives; at other times entire archives of solution-knowledges might be created and shared between people in different countries. The process is an enriching one for all who are involved. What a difference it can make to people to be joined with others in their struggles to address the problems of their lives.

Further Reading

Epston, D. & White, M. 1990: 'Consulting your consultants: The documentation of alternative knowledges'. *Dulwich Centre Newsletter*, No.4. Reprinted in Epston, D. & White, M. (1992): *Experience, Contradiction, Narrative & Imagination.* Adelaide: Dulwich Centre Publications.

Grieves, L. 1997: 'From beginning to start: The Vancouver Anti-Anorexia Anti-Bulimia League.' *Gecko,* Vol.2.

Madigan, S. & Epston, D. 1995: 'From "spy-chiatric gaze" to communities of concern: From professional monologue to dialogue.' In Friedman, S. (ed), *The Reflecting Team in Action* (pp.257-276). New York: Guilford. Reprinted in Epston, D. 1998: *Catching Up With David Epston: A collection of narrative practice-based papers.* Adelaide: Dulwich Centre Publications.

Nosworthy, S. & Lane, K. 1996: 'How we learnt that scratching can really be self-abuse: Co-research with young people.' *Dulwich Centre Newsletter,* No. 4.

Chapter 14

Outsider-witness groups and definitional ceremonies

Sometimes, narrative therapists create processes in which audience members act as witnesses, in very particular ways, to the conversations between the therapist and those coming to therapy. These processes are known as definitional ceremonies (after the work of Barbara Myerhoff, 1986). These can be powerful rituals in assisting people in the reclamation or redefinition of their identities.

The people who are recruited to be members of an audience to the conversation between the therapist and the person(s) consulting the therapist are often called outsider-witness groups. Sometimes outsider-witness groups are referred to as reflecting teams when this group is made up of professional colleagues.

Outsider-witness groups are made up of two or more people, either known or unknown to the person consulting the therapist. Outsider witnesses may be other therapists, family members, friends, members of a community or people unknown to the family, who may be able to offer some relevant expertise or experience. A child who has been subject to teasing and harassment may be interested in meeting with a team comprised of other children who have had a similar experience. Lesbian couples may be interested in outsider-witness groups comprising other members of the lesbian community. Aboriginal families or communities may choose to consult a team made up of some members of their community.

Narrative therapy often engages outsider-witness groups in a process (or definitional ceremony) that has four distinct stages. A room that is divided by a one-way screen is commonly used for these meetings, although this screen is not a necessity. When a screen is available, the therapist and person/family sit on one side of the screen, and the outsider-witness group sits behind the one-way mirror, listening to and watching the interview. In this way, the outsider-witness group cannot be seen by the family consulting the therapist, although family members know of and have approved of their presence. It is always up to the family members to decide whether or not they wish to have such a group as an audience to their conversations.

If a one-way screen is not available, the presence of one can be imagined. The separation this creates is important as it is more beneficial (and more ceremonial) if there is no interaction or dialogue, during the first three parts of the process, between the outsider-witness group on the one hand, and the therapist and family on the other. Outsider-witness groups have been used in many settings away from the 'traditional' therapy room, including within community gatherings (see further reading).

Part 1: Initial re-authoring conversation

The first part of the definitional ceremony involves the family and therapist joining in a re-authoring conversation. The outsider-witness group observes this conversation and listens carefully to what is being said.

Part 2: A retelling from the outsider-witness group

At the conclusion of the conversation between the therapist and the family, the outsider-witness group swaps places with them. The family is now behind the screen with the therapist and able to watch and listen as the outsider-witness group retells what they have just heard. The conversation between the members of the outsider-witness group is guided by the principles, ethics and practices of narrative therapy. Their retelling takes the form of a dialogue – questions and comments flow freely between the members of the group. These

retellings contribute to a rich description of the conversation that has just been witnessed.

They achieve this rich description by focusing on the emerging alternative stories of people's lives, and on the unique outcomes that were identified during Part 1 of the interview. Outsider-witness group members ask each other questions about anything that caught their attention, comment on events that they were curious about, and express curiosity about aspects of the conversation that they would like to understand more fully. Group members may also speculate on the meaning of certain events and hesitantly wonder about the implications of these for the future of the person/family consulting the therapist.

Alex, an outsider-witness group member might say: 'When Josie was talking I noticed she said that it was a relief to trust her mum with that piece of information. I was wondering more about what lead up to her being able to trust her mother like she did? And what that says about what Josie wants or is committed to in her relationship with her mother? I was wondering what this commitment might mean for their relationship and what Josie thinks about that?'

A smooth conversation amongst the members of the team is achieved by group members interviewing each other and by responding or adding to something that other group members have said. One member may say in response to Alex's comment: 'Yes, I was curious about the significance of Josie's trust in her mother also and I heard her mum say that their relationship is gaining closeness again. I wondered if it was a 'closeness' that Josie was committed to or maybe it is something else?'

Outsider-witness group members may then ask each other questions like: 'Why were you particularly interested in that? What did you hear that had you wondering about that event? Why do you think you are curious about that? What do you think that says about Josie and her mum's relationship that they are getting back their closeness?' The outsider-witness group members make it clear that they can only speculate about the family members' responses. Each time a speculation is entered into, it is done with the utmost of hesitancy and respect – team members never presume to know what is 'right' for the person or family. This is achieved through comments like, ' I'm not sure if this would fit with Josie, so I'd like to check it with her' or 'I'm not sure about that and would

really like to know more about it to make sure it would suit Josie and her relationships. I can't be certain about it but was just thinking that …'.

Group members also take care to explain why certain parts of the conversation caught their attention – perhaps because what they witnessed was similar to something that had occurred in their own lives, perhaps because it reminded them of someone or some event, or perhaps because it reflected something they had recently been reading of thinking about. Group members share the responsibility for recognising how what they have heard in some way resonates or connects with the experiences of their own lives, or with their own commitments and beliefs. In this way the hopes, commitments and beliefs of the outsider-witness group members become linked in some wáy with those of the family members. This can powerfully thicken the alternative stories of the lives of family members.

It is also usual for group members to talk about how the conversation they have witnessed has affected their thinking about their own lives or work, and/or its potential to shape and contribute to their lives or work practices in the future. This sharing is done in such a way that the family still remains at the centre of the retelling (as distinct from it being a personal sharing that centres the group members). This is known as de-centred sharing (White 1997). It is a deliberate and careful type of sharing, one that provides an acknowledgement of the ways in which the stories of the lives of the family members are linked to the stories of the lives of group members. It could sound something like this: 'When Josie was talking about trust, I was thinking about how I have sometimes had trouble finding trusting places in which to talk about certain things in my own life. Hearing Josie today has made me more conscious of how precious relationships of trust are. Her words will help me to think more about the people in my life whom I can trust and I will go away from here wanting to speak with them about what they mean to me.' Group members could then take this comment into a discussion by asking questions about it or by commenting on something they heard that had them thinking in similar ways.

In these contexts, attention to transparency (being open about why one is saying what one is saying) on behalf of the outsider-witness groups members is very important. Particular attention is also usually given to the difference in power between group members and the family in ways that minimise the potential for this imbalance to have harmful effects. Team members are careful to speak in

ways that recognise the family members as the experts on their own lives.

This conversation between outsider-witness group members continues until the allocated time is reached, or until the family members or the group members sense that it is time to swap places.

Part 3: The family member's response

The third part of this process provides an opportunity for the family members to comment on the retellings of the outsider-witness group. The therapist usually asks the family members about their responses to the retellings – for example, what they thought of the group's comments, what interested them about these comments, what did not interested them – and invites them to speak generally about the experience.

This part of the interview is not a continuation of the therapeutic conversation that occurred in Part 1. Instead, it is an opportunity for the family to comment on the retellings of the outsider-witness group and to have the last say on what was discussed. In this way, the group becomes more accountable to the family for the real effects of what they said – the group learns directly from the family members about what was most and least helpful to them. This feedback assists the group members in their further explorations of the practices of appropriate outsider-witness group retellings. Time is given for family members to give an account of their overall experience of being an audience to a conversation about their lives, and of how they predict this might affect their lives in the future.

Part 4: Discussion of the therapy

After the family members have commented on the retellings, the outsider-witness group is invited to join the therapist and the family. At this time there is an opportunity for everyone to reflect on the first three parts of the process.

The aim here is to invite everyone 'behind the scenes' of the therapy, thus making the therapeutic conversations transparent. The family members

may or may not wish to contribute to this discussion at this time. They may just listen. This practice of transparency fits with an ethical position held by many narrative therapists about only discussing the content of the interview or details of the life of the family members whilst the family is present.

The family and the outsider-witness group members are invited to ask the therapist anything about her/his contribution to the conversation. They might ask the therapist:

- what his/her thoughts were at certain points during the interview,

- why s/he asked particular questions,

- why s/he pursued one particular direction or 'line' of questions,

- what s/he thought about other options for the conversations during the interview,

- about 'turning points' in the interview,

- for clarification about any aspect of the therapeutic conversation that they wish to further understand,

- to speculate about the possibilities for future conversations with the family that may occur as a result of the meeting with the outsider-witness group.

During this fourth stage, the therapist may also interview the outsider-witness group members about their retellings, about their ideas on other possible questions that the family members could have been asked, and about they might have done if they had been taking the role of interviewer.

Summary

This chapter has described the four stages of the definitional ceremonies that are associated with narrative ways of working. When outsider-witness groups are used in community gatherings, or when they are made up of community members rather than professional workers, the process maybe modified. However the principles remain the same. The outsider-witness group is there to witness the re-authoring conversations and then to retell what they have heard in ways that contribute to rich description of alternative stories of

people's lives and identities.

People who consult therapists within the context of these definitional ceremonies invariably find this experience acknowledging and helpful. Family members say that hearing their stories in other people's words helps to further separate them from the problem-saturated stories of their lives, and contributes to profound developments in the rebuilding of their lives around preferred stories of their identity. Usually, families which have experienced the retellings of an outsider-witness group will specifically ask for this to be a part of their future consultations.

Further reading

'Reflecting teams.' 1999: Special edition of *Gecko*, Vol.2.

White, M. 1995: 'Reflecting team as definitional ceremony.' In White, M., *Re-authoring Lives: Interviews and essays,* chapter 7. Adelaide: Dulwich Centre Publications.

White, M. 1997: 'Definitional ceremony.' In White, M., *Narratives of Therapists' Lives,* chapter 4. Adelaide: Dulwich Centre Publications.

For examples of the use of outsider-witness groups in community gatherings, see:

'Reclaiming our stories, reclaiming our lives.' 1995: An initiative of the Aboriginal Health Council of South Australia. *Dulwich Centre Newsletter,* No.1.

'Speaking out and being heard,' 1995: *Dulwich Centre Newsletter,* No.4.

Closing remarks

This introductory book is now coming to a close and I am conscious of how much there is about narrative therapy that I haven't included in these pages. I have chosen not to discuss the broader theoretical ideas that locate narrative practices within the context of post-structuralist thought, and haven't described how literary theory and anthropology have influenced narrative practice. Instead I have tried to explain some of the key ideas. For this reason, I've deliberately used illustrations that are relatively uncomplicated. I hope that I have been able to convey the ideas without compromising their thoughtfulness or rigour.

To end, I thought I'd include a list of assumptions that inform narrative ways of working that I find very helpful to remind myself of every so often.

Assumptions that inform narrative ways of working:

❖ The problem is the problem (the person is not the problem).

❖ People have expertise on their own lives.

❖ People can become the primary authors of the stories of their own lives.

❖ By the time a person consults a therapist, they will have already made many attempts to reduce the influence of the problem in their lives and relationships.

❖ Problems are constructed in cultural contexts. These contexts include power relations of race, class, sexual preference, gender, and disadvantage.

❖ The problems for which people seek consultation usually cause them to reach thin conclusions about their lives and relationships. Often these conclusions have encouraged them to consider themselves as deficient in some way and this makes it difficult for them to access their knowledges,

competencies, skills and abilities.

❖ These skills, competencies and knowledges can be made available to them to assist with reclaiming their lives from the influence of the problem for which they seek help.

❖ There are always occasions in a person's life upon which they have escaped a problem's influence. Problems never successfully claim 100% of people's lives or relationships.

❖ Ensuring an atmosphere of curiosity, respect and transparency is the responsibility of the therapist.

References

Brigitte, Sue, Mem & Veronika, 1998: 'Power to our journeys.' In White, C. & Denborough, D. (eds), *Introducing Narrative Therapy: A collection of practice-based writings*. Adelaide: Dulwich Centre Publications.

Bruner, J. 1986: *Actual Minds: Possible worlds*. Cambridge, MA: Harvard University Press.

Freedman, J. & Combs, G. 1996: *Narrative Therapy: The social construction of preferred realities*. New York: Norton.

Geertz, C, 1973: 'Thick description: Toward an interpretative theory of culture.' In Geertz, C., *The Interpretation of Cultures*. New York: Basic Books.

Huntley, J. 1999: 'A narrative approach to working with students who have "learning difficulties".' In Morgan, A. (ed), *Once Upon a Time ... Narrative therapy with children and their families*. Adelaide: Dulwich Centre Publications.

Kamsler, A. 1990: 'Her-story in the making.' In Durrant, M. & White, C. (eds), *Ideas for Therapy With Sexual Abuse*. Adelaide: Dulwich Centre Publications. Reprinted 1998 in White, C. & Denborough, D. (eds), *Introducing Narrative Therapy: A collection of practice-based writings*. Adelaide: Dulwich Centre Publications.

Myerhoff, B. 1986: 'Life not death in Venice: Its second life.' In Turner, V. & Bruner, E. (eds), *The Anthropology of Experience*. Chicago: University of Illinois Press.

Myerhoff, B. 1982: 'Life history among the elderly: Performance, visibility and remembering.' In Ruby, J. (ed), *A Crack in the Mirror: Reflexive perspectives in anthropology*. Philadelphia: University of Pennsylvania Press.

Power to our journeys, 1999: 'Documents and treasures.' In Dulwich Centre Publications (ed), *Narrative Therapy and Community Work: A conference collection*. Adelaide: Dulwich Centre Publications.

Perry, L. 1999: 'There's a garden - somewhere.' In Morgan, A. (ed), *Once Upon a Time ... Narrative approaches with children and their families.* Adelaide: Dulwich Centre Publications.

Stiles, S, 1999: 'Community cultural development.' *Gecko,* Vol.3.

White, M. & Epston, D. 1990: *Narrative Means to Therapeutic Ends.* New York: Norton.

White, M. 1991: 'Deconstruction and therapy.' *Dulwich Centre Newsletter,* No.3. Reprinted in Epston, D. & White, M. (1992), *Experience, Contradiction, Narrative & Imagination.* Adelaide: Dulwich Centre Publications.

White, M, 1995: *Re-authoring Lives: Interviews & essays.* Adelaide: Dulwich Centre Publications.

White, M. 1997: *Narratives of Therapists' Lives.* Adelaide: Dulwich Centre Publications.

Index